PRAISE FOR *GUIDED BY DREAMS*

"*Guided by Dreams* is a sensational accomplishment. With clarity and insight, Rachel Norment explores the fascinating interface between the dreaming and waking worlds. This book offers a treasure chest of dreams that foretell both her illness and certain recovery. It is so well written, it reads like a novel! A must read for persons in the healing professions."

Stella Richards, Ph.D., psychologist and author of articles on psychology and early religious mythology, which regularly appear in *The San Francisco Jung Institute Library Journal.*

"Rachel Norment has written an important book for those who find themselves faced with the arresting diagnosis of breast cancer. This memoir while filled with a careful accounting of the author's experience contains invaluable information shared in a warm and deeply intimate conversational manner. If you or anyone you know has a diagnosis of breast cancer, this lovely book will surely become a guiding light."

Paula M. Reeves, Ph.D., psychotherapist and founder of *Spontaneous Contemplative Movement* and *Mindful Mirroring*; author of *Women's Intuition: Unlocking the Wisdom of the Body* and *Heart Sense: Unlocking Your Highest Purpose and Deepest Desires.*

"I like this book. I like the way Rachel takes us with her as she confronts the diagnosis of cancer, studies all the information she can, and then uses her dreams as guidance. We learn so much from what she learned. And, we are empowered by her example to trust our "inner healer," that part that "knows." I am especially thrilled that she introduces her readers to the Mandala Assessment Therapy, a method developed by art therapist Joan Kellogg, to accurately reveal the dynamics of our psyche. Some of her own drawings as she participated in Mandala Assessment are stunningly powerful. What Rachel did to heal, we can all do—in our own journey to wholeness."

P. M. H. Atwater, L.H.D.
Near-Death Researcher and author of many books, among them *The New Children and Near-Death Experiences* and *We Live Forever: The Real Truth About Death.*

"Everyone should read this book. It gives important information about prevention of illness, and can empower those facing any disease. The spiritual use of dreams can help us wake up more fully to the joy of being human."

Sandra McLanahan, M.D., and Co-author with David J. McLanahan of *Surgery and Its Alternatives*

Guided by Dreams

To Dee Dee,
May your dreams guide you in beneficial ways through your cancer experience — and all your life's journeys.
Best wishes!
Rachel 6/3/06

Guided by Dreams

Breast Cancer, Dreams, and Transformation

Rachel G. Norment

Rachel G. Norment

Foreword by Jeremy Taylor, D.Min.

Brandylane Publishers, Inc.
Richmond, Virginia

ISBN # 1-883911-66-4
Library of Congress Control Number: 2006922955

Brandylane Publishers, Inc.
Richmond, Virginia
www.brandylanepublishers.com

Some of the dreams discussed in this book have previously appeared and been interpreted in the author's columns, "Dreams" in the *Echo* (Charlottesville, Virginia) and "In Our Dreams" in the *Fluvanna Review*.

Cover Art: "Radiation Therapy" by Rachel Norment (see pages 98 & 99 for further details)

This book is lovingly dedicated to the memory of
my parents, Marcia Russell Gobbel
and Luther Lafayette Gobbel,
who instilled in me a love of the written word
and encouraged all my creative endeavors.

Contents

Foreword xiii

Preface xv

Acknowledgments xix

ONE - **When Trouble Strikes** 1

Holistic Approach to Health 4
Follow-up Mammogram & Scheduling Biopsy 6
The Biopsy 7
Awaiting Results of Biopsy 11
Getting the Results 13

TWO - **Seeking Counsel and Support** 18

Consultations with a Holistic Physician 20
Information from Friends 22
Conversation with a Pathologist and Holistic Physician 24
Sharing the News 26

THREE - **Taking Note of Dreams** 28

The Appointment with a Surgeon 32
Advice from a Surgeon Friend 36
Advice from an Intuitive Counselor 37
Questions Are Answered 40
Meeting a Radiation Oncologist 43

FOUR - **Facing the Knife** 48

Conversations with Other Breast Cancer Patients 49
Preparations for the Hospital Time 52
Pre-Admission Testing 53
A Puzzling Dream 53
Phone Consultation with My Surgeon 55
The Weekend Before Surgery 57

The Lumpectomy 57
Drainage Problems 62

FIVE - **Fearing the Fire** 69

Radiation Therapy 73
An Earlier Quest 79
Continuing Treatments 84

SIX - **Coping with Effects & Taking Precautions** 89

Discovering Hidden Emotions 101
Precautionary Measures 106
Homeopath 106
Essiac 108
Meeting Michael Lerner 119

SEVEN - **Discovering Contributing Factors** 121

Various Contributing Factors 125
Over-Mothering 126
Self-Nurture 128
Grief 131
Stress 133
Hormone Replacement Therap 147
Diet and Exercise 149

EIGHT-**Listening to Inner Wisdom** 153

Dreamwork Conference at Kanuga 158
A Difficult Dream to Interpret 163
Towards Transformatio 168

Epilogue 177
Appendix 184
Glossary 188
Bibliography 196
Author Bio 201

Dreams Contents By Titles

ONE - **When Trouble Strikes**
Medical Tests with a Tube Inserted 7
Microscopic Organisms Enter My Skin 12

TWO - **Seeking Counsel and Support**

THREE - **Taking Note of Dreams**
I Fear the Woman is Drowning 28
The Short Man Easily and Gently Carries Me 29
I Choose to Stay In and Rest 29
I Go into the Men's Room 29
I Dump the Excrement into a Man's Cap 30
The Man Wants Me to Participate in His Group 30
The Man Avoids Me; My Friend Goes On Ahead of Me 39

FOUR - **Facing the Knife**
From Burning Coals to a Fountain 54

FIVE - **Fearing the Fire**
The Woman Denies Having Breast Cancer 75

SIX - **Coping with Effects & Taking Precautions**
I Dig Up a Shoulder and Breas 102
A Family Consultation with a Doctor 103
Fighting for My Life 104
A Flesh-Eating Toxin 105
The Instructor Sends Me to Get a Drink 110
The Game of Forced Combat 111
The Instructor Doesn't Respect My Desire for Privacy 115
I Don't Want to Sleep in Bed Full of Fleas 116
I Have On the Wrong Color Robe 117
I Want to Sweep Away the Dead Bugs 118

SEVEN - **Discovering Contributing Factors**
Picking Up a Copperhead 121
Another Snake Bite 123

Being Aware of a Snake Near Our Path 124
A Commode Morphs into a Spa Tub 129
The Teacher Takes Care of My Kitten 130
I Show My Mother a Kitten 131
I Need to Take Care of the Motherless Kitten 131
I Fear the Fire Will Spread Beyond the Contained Area 133
I Go into the Men's Room 136
I Need Peace and Quiet 137
I Lament Our Crowded Living Conditions 138
I Search for My Assigned Space 138
I Want Only My Things in My Suitcase 140
I Fear Animals and Humans Outside Our Tower Priso 141
Trying to Escape an Institution 142
I Obey Authorities Against My Mother's Advice 144
No Longer Will the Woman Hide from Authorities 146
I Will Accept the Role of Doctor 150

EIGHT-**Listening to Inner Wisdom**
Large Insects Are Damaging Our Room 154
My Kitten's Strange Growth Needs to Be Cut Off 155
A Growth on My Neck Needs to Be Removed 155
I Worry about Dangerous Growths in Our House 156
Being Examined While on a Hospital Gurney 157
Medical Tests with a Tube Inserted 157
The Kitten Needs Nourishment and Loving Care 158
From Burning Coals to a Fountain 160
The Man Wants Me to Participate in His Group 162
I Choose to Stay In and Rest 163
I Dump the Excrement into a Man's Cap 164
I Observe Progress in the Rejuvenation of My Future Home 165
I Proudly Watch the Renovation of My Old House 167
I Want to Be Told What to Teach 170
My Large Cat Speaks 173
The Cat Speaks in a Human Voice 174
I Have On the Wrong Color Robe 176

Epilogue

I Must Keep Checking the Contents of a Container 177
A Head to Care For 178
Babies with Just Heads 179
A Man's Bald Head in a Box 180
I Meet a Very Special Woman 181
I Am to Give a Life-Saving Demo or Lecture to Wome 182

Foreword

I have known Rachel Norment for many years. When we meet, we always share the chapter in our evolving creative, spiritual journeys. We also share and explore dreams together, in depth, on these occasions. Our connections have deepened in this process and we have become friends. When, Nancy, my step-mother, died, it was not from my half-siblings, but from Rachel that I first heard the news.

The book that you hold in your hand is a poignant record of Rachel's interior and external life during her successful battle with cancer. She shares her experiences with candor and grace, and gives us glimpses into the subtle interior, emotional process, as well as careful account of the external struggle of one unusually conscious, intelligent, creative, and courageous woman dealing with the "shadow of death" as it fell across her life path, a deeply personal path she also walks with her partner and life's companion, Owen.

My professional specialty is exploring and trying to understand more about the deeper meanings of the dreams we all have, every night, and sometimes remember when we wake. Rachel is generous in sharing her dreams on these pages. Remembering and working to understand the multiple meanings of her dreams is a central part of her evolving drama of healing. It is both moving and fascinating to see how her thoughts and feelings have deepened and developed over time, from the initial experiences in response to her diagnosis, through the process of deciding what measures to take to help the body heal itself, to the even more developed reflections shared in this book.

Like all dreams, the dreams she shares with us here are spontaneous symbolic reflections of the deeper truth of interior life and external experience. At the universal, archetypal level, her dreams, just like all our dreams, speak for themselves, always telling more about us and our lives than we realize consciously when we are awake.

Dreams speak a universal language of metaphor and symbol. (Carl Jung called these repeating patterns of meaning and significance "archetypes of the collective unconscious.") Another great truth about dreams and dream narratives is that they always carry many different levels of meaning and significance simultaneously, like emotionally charged, symbol laden puns. The dreamer's own comments and understandings are always the most important part of the larger, more complex and multi-layered truth that the dreams convey, and at the same time, there are always more layers than the dreamer can see easily without the help of others.

Rachel offers many insights reflecting her healing and her own growing understandings of her dreams during this emotionally turbulent and demanding period of her life. She tells us some of how they reflect and offer gentle guidance in her on-going efforts to heal her body, and go on living and loving in the face of cancer. These dreams and the precious insights they provided are offered to us with tremendous generosity and care.

This book is also illustrated with some of the drawings and paintings that flowed from Rachel's hands as she grounded her emotional efforts in concrete, ongoing creative meditations. These wonderful images are an integral part of the narrative and document the healing process in the same poignant, symbolic fashion as the dreams themselves. The pictures also invite us to follow Rachel on her path of healing and spiritual development. Rachel models and offers us creative ways of discovering and enriching our own journeys of self-healing and spiritual development.

There is much wisdom and startling beauty in this book. May you all enjoy and profit from this book as much as I have.

Reverend Jeremy Taylor, D.Min.

—Co-founder and past president of the International Association of the Study of Dreams and author of *Dream Work, Where People Fly and Water Runs Up Hill*, and *The Living Labyrinth*

Preface

For many years I have been compelled to seek answers through reading whatever appropriate material I can find on my current subject of concern. I am convinced that I am being led, by a Higher Source, to find the books I need at any given time. When I go to a bookstore I usually browse in a section of my current interest to see what is available. Frequently one or two books catch my eye. Sometimes a book I have glanced at and then put back on the shelf at an earlier time now seems to be the one I should read.

When I learned that I had breast cancer, I immediately went to a bookstore and came home with five or six books relating to cancer, some with medical information, others relating personal experiences of patients. One of the first I read was *First You Cry* by Betty Rollin. I found it very helpful to know someone else's personal experiences while going through cancer treatments, and decided to keep a daily journal of my own experiences, thinking that perhaps some day what I experienced and learned might help someone else. I recorded the events of the day, including actual conversations, into my journal the day they were happening. I wanted to have a true record of what was happening and the information I was receiving. Therefore, I have not added any fictional embellishments in this account.

My interest in dreams extends back at least thirty years. I kept a dream journal briefly in 1972, but during the subsequent twenty years, my time was mainly filled with raising two children along with becoming a professional artist exhibiting in area, regional, and national exhibitions, and teaching art classes first for a community college, then privately. In 1992 I became serious in my efforts to record dreams daily, or as frequently as I remembered any. I attended my first dreamwork workshop, "Dreams and Healing," at the Institute of Higher Healing in Richmond, Virginia, on February 22, 1992. It was conducted by psychologist John Windsor and Joan Windsor (author of *The Inner Eye, Dreams and Healing, Passages of Light,* and *Dreamwork).* I was amazed to discover that one could understand the symbolism of dreams and I wanted to learn more, so I began reading available books on the subject.

The evening following my cancer diagnosis I asked my

unconscious (my inner or Higher Self) to give me some information about my situation through a dream. I did not remember any dream the next two mornings, but on the third morning I recalled a series of six dreams. The first dream seemed to state by means of metaphors what had already happened. I could not immediately understand the rest. I gradually realized the second dream was helping me make a decision concerning my course of treatment. The remaining dreams contributed information in a variety of ways—two of them foretelling future events.

My experience with breast cancer proved not to be the horror story that many have had to go through. I was fortunate that the prognosis for the kind of cancer I had was good. Nevertheless any cancer diagnosis is serious and the experience was certainly traumatic while it was happening.

This book recounts in detail my experiences, thoughts, and emotions surrounding my diagnosis and treatments, and how I used the knowledge gained through dream interpretation to make decisions during the course of my treatment and in the years immediately following. Thereby, I hope to make the reader aware that there may be multiple options for one to consider when faced with such a traumatic illness. By revealing my thoughts and emotions, I hope to show those faced with a cancer diagnosis that others understand firsthand what they are going through.

Dreams have many layers. I deal with several layers of some of the dreams; of others I deal with only the meanings that were conscious in my thinking at the time of the experience or with the meaning that best illustrates a point I wish to make. Sometimes understanding even a simple meaning was slow in coming. Sometimes I learned a meaning too late to actually help during decision making. I wish I had been more experienced at interpreting my dreams at that time. In fact, had I been more cognizant of the meaning of dreams several years before my diagnosis I might have understood several warnings. But I was not delving very deeply, if at all, into the interpretation of those early dreams. Then too, I forgot about most of them until years later when I began reviewing the early dreams to see whether there had been any warnings. Some things are clearly seen and understood only in hindsight. This was certainly true in my case.

My illness and efforts to understand what my dreams were

trying to tell me about the illness and its causes and possible treatments became a powerful learning experience. I came to realize that the whole experience was a "wake-up call"—a life-transforming event—part of my education, my preparation for my life's purpose. In 1991, three years before the cancer was diagnosed, I consciously began asking myself what more am I supposed to do with my life beyond being a wife, mother, artist, and teacher. One might think this is enough, but I began to feel that it wasn't. Some of my dreams since then reveal that my quest followed an inner plan for me, incorporating a new direction—one that is now unfolding.

Through this experience and guidance from my inner or Higher Self as revealed by dreams, I have experienced an awakening to Feminine Spirituality, the same awakening that Sue Monk Kidd describes in *The Dance of the Dissident Daughter*. When I read her book recently, having already written several drafts of this manuscript, I resonated with her experience; it sounded very familiar to me. An understanding of deeper levels of my dreams—many presented in this book plus many others—reveal this awakening.

Wanting to become proficient in understanding my dreams, during the past decade I have taken the opportunity whenever possible to attend workshops and seminars led by nationally and internationally known dreamworkers, including Wallace and Jean Clift, James Hollis, Robert Johnson, Stanley Krippner, Julia McAfee, Paula Reeves, Angelo Spoto, Murray Stein, Jeremy Taylor, Montague Ullman, Barry Williams, and Marion Woodman. I have learned so much from these enlightened, discerning counselors and teachers about human nature and dreams.

To use an expression I learned from Jeremy Taylor, I believe that "all dreams come to us in the service of health and wholeness." We can receive warnings of impending health problems and advice on possible courses of treatment that may lead to physical cures, but even if we are not "cured" in the medical sense, we may be "healed"—be made whole. Dreams can help us become *conscious* psychologically in order to become fully the person we are meant to become. After becoming aware of many previously "hidden" aspects of ourselves, we can integrate these with those already in our consciousness, thus becoming more nearly whole individuals.

In order to benefit from our dreams we must first pay attention to them and record them for future reference. We also need to learn how to interpret them. I hope that my story will encourage you to become more aware of the importance of dreams, to begin recording your own dreams, and to learn how to understand them. The sooner you begin, the sooner you will be able to benefit from them. They can help you make decisions about treatments if you become ill. By listening to what dreams tell you is important, you might also understand what could become the source of a potential illness. By taking appropriate action after understanding a dream, you might even be able to prevent an illness. Dreams can help you know yourself more fully and lead you in discovering your life's purpose.

May this book inspire you to let dreams be your guides.

Acknowledgments

I am profoundly grateful to the physicians and counselors whose skills, knowledge, and compassionate care helped me to successfully make my way through very stressful times: Dr. Richard Belgrad, Dr. Mitchell Fleisher, Dr. Shelton Horsley, Dr. Sandra McLanahan, Dr. Anthony Munoz, Dr. Eric Swensson, Dr. Vernon Sylvest, and Joan Windsor. I am also pleased that each one has given permission to be called by their own names in this book, thus enabling me to publicly thank them. The names of various other persons have been changed to give them anonymity.

I wish to thank all the unnamed friends who offered encouragement and showed they cared by driving me to treatments in Richmond, providing meals, and giving beautiful flowers to add beauty to my surroundings during the experience recounted in this book. These expressions of love and concern lessened the trauma of the time.

I am grateful to Jeremy Taylor for his many contributions towards this book. His insights about some of my dreams, offered at workshops I attended through the years, helped immensely, as have comments and suggestions regarding the manuscript. I give special thanks for a wonderful foreword and for his friendship. He is an inspiration to me and countless others as we endeavor to learn how to understand and be guided by our dreams.

I am indebted to Morgan Simone Daleo and Kathleen Phalen who taught courses in Memoir Writing and Creative Nonfiction that helped me gain enough writing skills to undertake this project. Morgan was the first person to read the initial draft. Her encouragement and advice were greatly appreciated.

I am grateful to many additional people who gave generously of their time to read the manuscript in its early stages, then offered comments of encouragement and suggestions for its improvement: P.M.H. Atwater, Eleanor Kratter, Sandra McLanahan, Paula Reeves, Stella Richards, Grace Silverman, and Patty Wallens.

I owe many thanks to the workshop and seminar leaders whom I name in my preface. I have learned so much from each one.

I am indebted to many too numerous to name, literally a couple of hundred authors, whose books on dreamwork, symbolism, and mythology line my shelves and have provided helpful insights into dream interpretation.

I thank Robert Pruett of Brandylane Publishers, Inc., for accepting my book and providing skillful editing, enthusiastic support, and warm encouragement. I appreciate all he and his staff have done to successfully bring this new creation into the world.

I am blessed with a wonderful daughter and son, Marcia and Russell. Their love and support through this experience helped immensely, as did that from my brother, Russell Gobbel, and his family.

Most of all, I want to thank my husband, Owen, for his special love and emotional support throughout our many decades together and especially during this traumatic experience. In addition, I owe him thanks for his skilled editorial help in fine-tuning this manuscript and his ongoing help in mundane household matters, allowing me extra time to follow my creative passions and dreams.

1

When Trouble Strikes

> Diseases can be our spiritual flat tires—disruptions in our lives that seem to be disasters at the time, but end by redirecting our lives in a meaningful way.
>
> — Bernie S. Siegel, M.D.

I assumed my routine mammogram would turn out like many I had had before. But I was mistaken. On Friday, June 11, 1993 I went for the mammogram at the Breast Center of Chippenham Hospital in Richmond, Virginia—just a little over a year since the previous one. I had been getting a mammogram each year for many years. After going through the usual routine of waiting to see if the x-rays "took," I was sent home, assured I would be notified about the results.

The following Monday I received a phone call. "Mrs. Norment, the doctor wants you to return to have more mammograms done." "Why?" I questioned. "What is the problem?"

The person calling could not tell me why this was necessary. "Well, when I come back in, will I be able to know before I leave the hospital what they find this time?" I questioned further. "I don't want to have to wait again to know what's going on." "Yes, we'll let you know before you leave."

This call really worried me. In the past, hearing nothing verbally, I would assume everything was okay. I would receive an official notice: "Your recent mammogram did not show any sign of cancer. A copy of your report has been forwarded to your physician." The only problem was that sometimes it would be four to six weeks before I would receive the notice. I would laugh at the reference to "recent" mammogram. My connotation of "recent" evidently is different from theirs.

Why would they want me to come all the way back into

Richmond, an hour and a half drive from my home at Hampden-Sydney (a small college community in southside Virginia, where my husband Owen, a Presbyterian minister, was Professor of Religion until his retirement in 1998)? Didn't they take enough mammograms while I was there on Friday? They took the usual number. I have always had lots of fibrous tissue in my breasts, which I have understood is common in many women and doesn't necessarily indicate the presence of a tumor. I recalled that ten or fifteen years earlier one doctor had been concerned after breast palpation and sent me to someone else to be checked further. At that time my imagination ran wild. I might have breast cancer. What would it be like to have it? Fortunately, this proved to be a false alarm. Nothing was wrong.

When I returned to the Breast Center on Tuesday, I questioned why more mammograms were needed. The nurse technician said something about "not being sure of the film, needing clarification." Again I went through the whole procedure.

Despite being previously promised I'd be told the results of the x-ray before I left the hospital, upon completion of the session I was informed that the radiologist was not there; I would have to wait to be notified. Didn't they know the radiologist wouldn't be there when I talked to them over the phone setting up the new appointment? Another wait!

The doctor was supposed to call me the next morning. By afternoon, still not having heard and getting too anxious to wait any longer, I called. After a long wait holding the phone, I finally was put through.

The radiologist seemed very concerned. "Mrs. Norment," she began. "Something is showing up on your left breast, but I can't tell what it might be. The mammogram shows a new small density on one view only, the flat up and down compression. One dimension is less than a centimeter (less than 1/2 inch) and the other four millimeters. I think it is too small to be felt by hand examination. I don't think it would show up on ultrasound. On the second take, it appeared to be smaller, but it did not go away." "Well, what do you think it is?" "It doesn't look suspicious; it doesn't look like a cyst," she replied. "We can't tell exactly where in the breast mass it is since it showed up only in one view. It must be hidden behind white breast tissue in other views. I recommend a needle biopsy, which is done under mammogram and with a local anesthetic."

She mentioned something about a needle attachment to the mammogram machine that would lead a surgeon to where he needed to go. At least this was what I thought she was saying. Being unfamiliar with this procedure, I was puzzled and wondered what she meant. Was it something that would be left in my breast between the needle biopsy and surgery? She listed other options: "One, to continue watching with mammograms. Two, surgical biopsy under local anesthetic." It seemed that she was saying there were two different kinds of biopsy.

"I recommend you get an appointment with a surgeon to see if he feels a biopsy should be done," she advised. With this our conversation ended.

By this time I was very concerned and confused. I felt I should talk with my gynecologist and a surgeon before deciding what to do. When I called my gynecologist I asked two questions.

"How does this differ from fibrous breast tissue that has been seen on my mammograms for years?"

Her answer was simply, "It could be this [fibrous tissue]."

"I don't understand completely about the needle attachment to lead the surgeon to the site. Is this for the needle biopsy or surgical biopsy?" I asked.

She informed me that with the aid of x-rays (Does she mean more mammograms?) the "marker" is put in. I'm not sure whether I learned the details of the full process at this time, but as I learned later, a needle is inserted into the breast down to the area in question. Mammograms are taken several times during the process to be sure the needle goes to the right place. Next, a wire is inserted through the needle, then the needle is removed, leaving the wire in place. This is left there to guide the surgeon who will either excise the lump or aspirate it. She then recommended I call Dr. Erik Swensson, surgeon.

I felt the need for additional advice from someone whose judgment I trusted. I called Dr. Vernon Sylvest to ask his opinion. At the time Dr. Sylvest was Medical Director of the Roche Biomedical Laboratories (which subsequently merged with Laboratory Corporation of America). I had known him in his role as Director of the Institute of Higher Healing in Richmond, Virginia. Also, I knew his own inspiring story of healing (subsequently published in 1997 as *The Formula)* and his holistic approach in medicine. After hearing my recitation of what had been happening, he recommended a needle biopsy and the surgeon Erik Swensson, whom he referred to as his friend, thus confirming my doctor's recommendations.

I followed through with an appointment with Dr. Swensson the following Monday. Owen, my concerned husband, drove me to Richmond. After a wait in the large, neatly appointed waiting room of the Richmond Surgical Associates, I was shown the way back to an examining room. After another wait, Swensson, a tall, handsome man with dark hair, came in followed by a nurse. He shook my hand, greeted me pleasantly, and proceeded to examine my breasts, palpating them carefully trying to see if he could feel any mass.

Having already viewed my mammograms, he announced, "I can't tell what is there. It might just be overlapping tissue. It would be very difficult to do a biopsy since it is not visible in the second view. I wouldn't know where to aim. I recommend you wait and have more mammograms in six months." "Can we get Owen back here? I'd like you to show us the place in question on the mammograms," I asked.

Owen was summoned from the waiting room and Dr. Swensson patiently pointed out the area in question. He reeled off a bunch of statistics on the chances of this being cancer. What stuck in my mind was that only 20 % of suspicious tumors might be malignant, so we could rest relatively assured that this wasn't anything serious. We were relieved and I actually put any related concern out of my mind for the next six months.

HOLISTIC APPROACH TO HEALTH

> This concept, holistic medicine, is, for the first time in our history, an integration of the two approaches [the "allopathic" and "naturopathic" views], taking the best from each and using them in conjunction to potentiate each other.
>
> —Lawrence LeShan,
> *Cancer as a Turning Point*

On July 1, 1993, eleven days after the first visit to the surgeon, I had my first appointment with Dr. Sandra McLanahan, a capable family physician specializing in complementary and integrative medicine, and co-author with her brother, David J. McLanahan, M.D., of the comprehensive volume *Surgery and Its Alternatives* (2002). I first heard of her several years earlier, but it took me this long to decide that I should go to her. Dr. McLanahan's home base is in Yogaville at the Satchidananda Ashram, a spiritual center situated on the banks of the James River south of Scottsville, Virginia. In addition to being the Executive Medical Director of the Integral Health Center there and periodically assisting Dr. Dean Ornish with programs and research in California, she was seeing some patients at the Institute of Higher Healing in Richmond, Virginia, when I first went to her.

There were various facets of my health I thought needed attention. For at least eight years I had been taking allergy shots, fighting respiratory allergies. I also puzzled over what foods might be causing problems. Off and on over the years I have experienced vaginal yeast infections, sometimes painful. I had also been counseled to make an effort to bring my cholesterol down. Since 1987 I had been on Hormone Replacement Therapy (HRT), a combination of Premarin and Progesterone, which was causing me to have monthly periods even though I was post-menopausal. I was annoyed with this, and concerned that HRT might eventually cause other problems, I wanted to discontinue it. Then too, I knew I needed to find a way to lose weight.

Sandra McLanahan gave me a thorough exam, checking out the color and texture of my skin and nails as well as the usual examination of ears, eyes, and heart beat. She felt that my immune system was quite depressed. Having assisted Dr. Dean Ornish for years in doing research and teaching patients, she follows the holistic approach to health that he advocates in his nationally known program for the reversal of heart disease: low fat, high complex carbohydrate diet; aerobic exercises; yoga, meditation, vitamins and herbal supplements, homeopathic remedies, and relaxation techniques.

Owen (who began seeing Sandra two weeks later) and I began following the program. I needed to follow a more limited diet than he did, but he graciously volunteered to help me learn how to cook differently. The change in diet proved to be quite a challenge. We were very frustrated during the first weeks and months learning menus and recipes. We were not supposed to use any added fats or sugars. I was not allowed any bread, except rice crackers and pita, and no chicken or beef for the next three months. We both began losing weight. I was losing at the rate of a pound a week. We were delighted and felt we were on the right path.

> The problem is not the existence or nonexistence of the individual's self-healing powers, but in how to mobilize them and bring them into play in the person's search for health.
>
> — Lawrence LeShan,
> *Cancer as a Turning Point*

FOLLOW-UP MAMMOGRAM AND SCHEDULING BIOPSY

On Wednesday, December 15, 1993, I returned for the follow-up mammograms. The technician took several views of just the left breast, deciding the right breast did not need to be x-rayed at this time. I waited while the film was developed and the radiologist reviewed them, then the nurse ushered me into the radiologist's office.

"Mrs. Norment," the doctor began in a concerned voice. "Something is definitely visible in two views. But it has not gotten any bigger than it was back in June. I recommend that you have a biopsy. You should get another appointment with your surgeon." With this she handed me a booklet on breast disease, including cancer. Now I had real reason to worry.

Due to the Christmas season and the doctor's vacation I had to wait until Tuesday, January 4, 1994, for an appointment with Dr. Swensson. After viewing the mammograms, he stated I should have a needle localization biopsy. He tried to be optimistic, stating the statistics that 80% to 90% of potential problems turn out to be benign. We scheduled a biopsy for Tuesday, January 18, two weeks away.

Owen made a reservation for Monday night, January 17, at a hotel located near Johnston-Willis Hospital, where the procedure was to be done. But the day before my scheduled biopsy, faced with the possibility of an ice storm, we wondered if it would be possible to get to Richmond. When the storm materialized, my surgery was rescheduled for the following Tuesday. This extended the time between my visit with the surgeon on January 4 and the biopsy to three weeks. Tensions within me began to build.

On Saturday we received a call from a member of the Burkeville Presbyterian Church, where Owen was preaching once a month, to tell us of the death of a member. We had attended a Christmas Open House at the now deceased woman's home. A week or so after that occasion she told Owen she had a recurrence of cancer and was not given long to live. Her funeral was to be held on Sunday afternoon.

I went with Owen, but I found it emotionally difficult. When we arrived at the cemetery I told Owen to go on over to the grave site, where other ministers were already waiting for him. Even though I had not yet had the biopsy and did not want to believe I could possibly have breast cancer, subconsciously I felt something was wrong. I didn't want to walk into the cemetery. I wanted to run away, drive off in the opposite direction. But I managed to pull myself together, dried my tears, and went over to the grave site for the funeral.

THE BIOPSY

A dream which occurred almost a year and a half earlier, on October 3, 1992, should be mentioned here.

Medical Tests with a Tube Inserted

Others and I are undergoing some kind of "tests" which seem to be medical. We are being anesthetized to have some "tube" or something inserted. This will be left in so the results can be observed and recorded.

At the time I had no idea what this dream could mean. It's the kind of dream you are tempted not to record because you remember so little and you can't see its significance. Only long after receiving my cancer diagnosis and completing treatments did I even recall having this dream. I was amazed to realize it might have been foretelling an event I would experience much later, a procedure I knew nothing about at the time.

On Monday, January 24, 1994, the weather allowed us to go to Richmond without any problem. We stayed at the hotel as we had originally planned. After having supper at a nearby restaurant, we went to see the film *Shadowland* about C. S. Lewis and his wife, who died of cancer. What a choice. It was a very moving film, but a difficult story to be viewing right before a biopsy.

Before going to sleep, using my Walkman I played a tape I made reading some visualizations and affirmations with background music. I woke up several times during the night aware of noise and the chatter of people going in and out by the front desk area, our room being very near the front lobby. But I managed to go back to sleep each time.

Arriving at Johnston-Willis by 6:50 a.m., I went directly into Radiology to have the numbing cream put on the skin at the spot where the needle would be inserted, in order to allow time for the cream to take effect. Then I went out to the Outpatient Surgery desk to officially register.

Back in Radiology, I watched a brief video on breast cancer. By this time I was very nervous and broke into tears. I managed to compose myself as I was called into the mammography room where the needle and wire were to be inserted. I didn't want to be crying as I walked into the room. I knew it was important for me to remain calm and composed while undergoing the procedure. Seeing how nervous I was, the nurse called in a volunteer to be there with me.

My breast was compressed by the mammogram apparatus using a plastic plate with holes through which the needle could be inserted. The radiologist inserted the needle. Mammograms were taken periodically during the procedure to see if the needle was going to the spot where the lesion was. A wire was inserted through the needle and left in place after the needle was removed. This wire would guide the surgeon's knife during the actual biopsy.

Before the procedure began I was asked to remove my clothes, including my shoes. Since I'm sensitive to cold—especially in over-air-conditioned places—I wanted to leave my shoes on. It helps me feel warm if I keep my feet warm. I was told that, no, I needed to take them off. A little later I saw why. Blood ran down onto my knees and then to the floor. It did miss my feet though. Had it not and had I left my shoes on, they would have been a mess.

I was amazed there was no pain during this part of the procedure. As I had been told, the skin must be the most sensitive part of the breast. With the wire in place, I was asked to get on a gurney where they covered me with blankets to keep me warm, then wheeled me back to the pre-operation waiting cubicle.

A nurse who came in to make preparations seemed confused about what she needed to be doing. I asked if I would be given an antibiotic. Since at the time it was thought that my heart had a midsystolic click (a kind of murmur), doctors had advised giving an antibiotic to prevent infection during surgery. The nurse checked my chart and said yes, there were instructions to give this. After getting the drip bag apparatus, she inserted the IV needle into a vein in my right hand and started the antibiotic.

The insertion of the wire had been completed by 9:00 a.m. An hour later I was still waiting in the cubicle. Owen was brought back and waited with me until after Dr. Swensson came back to see me. Swensson had been delayed in OR with another operation longer than anticipated. He said my operation would begin soon. I was told that they were cleaning up the OR to get ready for me. I think I waited another twenty minutes or so.

Finally sometime around 11:00 a.m. I was wheeled into OR. I decided I didn't want anything to make me drowsy. I had gotten over most of my nervousness and I figured I could manage with just the local anesthetic. I was moved from the gurney to the operating table and covered with a blanket. All the nurses by this time were aware I was cold. They kept making apologies. The room was very cold. They said the theory was the germs didn't like the cold. At the time I thought this made sense—freezing the germs would kill them. On reflection, maybe they were making a joke, since it clearly was not cold enough to freeze the germs.

Grounding plates were placed on my thighs, as a precaution, since cauterization would be used. My arms were placed on board extensions and straps were placed around my arms and legs to remind me not to move. My breast was painted with what I took to be a brown antiseptic soap. A small clip was attached to my right thumb to monitor the amount of oxygen in my blood. A blood pressure cuff was attached to my right arm.

After Dr. Swensson came in, they put up a "tent" over my head as a screen between my eyes and what was being done. In a way, to satisfy my curiosity, I might have liked being able to see what was going on, but watching the actual procedure might have been upsetting. In a kind voice Dr. Swensson said, "I'll explain everything I do. If you have pain, let me know." Later he asked if I was feeling any pain. At one point, when I said it was stinging some, they injected a little more anesthetic.

I heard another male voice speak with Swensson. I heard Swensson say, "There it is." I assumed he had found the lesion. I also thought I heard him give the instruction "No frozen section." I wondered what would be discovered. Was it cancer?

Swensson said they would be finishing up soon. But it seemed to me to be quite some time before they were ready to do the stitches. I felt lots of tugging and heard what I assume was suctioning of fluids. I feared I was bleeding more than expected. At a consultation with Dr. Swensson several weeks later I asked him if I had bled more than usual. "No," he replied. "Sometimes it takes fifteen minutes to clear out all the fluids from one small area. I wanted to leave the area absolutely dry, so I continued for as long as necessary to do so."

Dr. Swensson told me before he left OR that he would call me in a couple of days if there was a problem. Otherwise he would see me in a week to remove the stitches.

A nurse told me that the incision was quite small, requiring only three stitches. A bandage was placed over the wound and a clear tape sealed the outer edges. I was transferred back to the gurney and was wheeled into the recovery room. There the nurse monitored my blood pressure, took my temperature, and asked if I felt okay. Fairly soon I was allowed to dress and walk out to the waiting room.

Owen was surprised by my arrival. He was anxious, wondering what was happening. One of the nurses had told us before my surgery that Dr. Swensson would come out to talk with him after finishing the operation. When he didn't appear, Owen feared the operation was still going on all the time I was in the recovery room.

Although I felt very little discomfort from the surgery, after lunch, when my breast began to hurt some, we stopped at a drug store to buy some Tylenol.

AWAITING RESULTS OF BIOPSY

Following the biopsy, we had another week-long wait. After a couple of days I became acutely aware of the incoming phone calls. Owen said it was unfortunate that Swensson had left it the way he did because we would be fearful that every phone call was bad news. It would have been better had he intended to call no matter what. He did not call all weekend. Owen tried to be encouraging, saying that it meant everything was okay. But I had a feeling the doctor might be waiting until I came on Tuesday to tell us anything, not wanting to give bad news over the phone.

Days earlier when I was discussing with his secretary the appointment timing she suggested it might be good to have a friend come with me if Owen couldn't come. From this I sensed that she felt he might be telling me bad news. I speculated that maybe he had a habit of waiting until the follow-up appointment to tell the bad news.

During this next weekend, while waiting to hear the diagnosis from the doctor, I decided to sit at my drawing table and paint. For the past twenty-some years painting had been a major part of my life. I had gradually focussed on watercolor as my primary medium and had achieved considerable success and recognition as a watercolor artist. Using a full sheet (22" x 30") of watercolor paper, I began to paint spontaneously, without thought of what I would paint. I was not pleased with the result; I thought it was awful. What I first thought of as an abstract design on closer inspection looked like a huge erupting volcano. I did not think the painting was worth saving. I certainly wouldn't show it anywhere. I disliked it so much I took scissors and cut it into four pieces—neatly, into exact fourths. You might think I would have crumpled it up and thrown it away, but for some unexplainable, unconscious reason I didn't; I put it away in my art cabinet. Looking at it many months later, I realized it is the perfect metaphor for the state of my mind at that time. I'm glad I saved it. It shows the fear, terror building inside me, ready to explode while I was waiting for the diagnosis.

In my recent reading on dream interpretation I was struck by a comment by Marc Ian Barasch in his insightful book, *Healing Dreams.* He states that "[c]ancer might be represented as a landscape swarming with insect plague, or by lava-spewing volcano." My spontaneous painting was not of a dream, but it came from the same place that dreams come from—my unconscious mind, the part of myself that is beneath the level of conscious awareness. So the painting—now entitled *Emotions*—was, indeed, a perfect metaphor for my anxious state of mind while waiting for the diagnosis. It may be found on page 93.

The first metaphor suggested in Barasch's statement reminded me of a dream I had on Wednesday, June 16, 1993, the night before receiving the results on the mammogram first showing a suspicious spot. Part of the lengthy dream states:

Microscopic Organisms Enter My Skin

I have been observing something strange going on in my body. Somewhere on my skin there is a place where there may be an almost microscopic opening where microscopic organisms are entering. I look at it and wonder what might be going on. But I can't really tell and then I can't really see anything and I don't think further about it. On the following day . . . I observe this place again. (It may have been on a breast, but the place was not specified in the dream. I know it wasn't labeled left breast in the dream.) This time I see something microscopic crawling into this pore-like place. I may begin to squeeze it like you do with a blackhead. After a few seconds or minutes I see a thin string-like substance begin to come out the tiny opening. It continues 'till a string of white substance one to two inches long has come out. Then I squeeze a little more and I see a larger white something begin to push the opening wider and finally the whole thing pops out. . . . I catch it with my fingers and put it on a Kleenex. I am relieved to know what the strange place on the skin has been about and that it is nothing of consequence and that it is out. I go looking for Owen to show him . . . . I am relieved to know what is going on and it is not a further problem.

At the time I wondered if this meant I would receive the same good news about my breast or if it was just wishful thinking. Later in the day, I was told by the radiologist that there was a new small density showing on the mammogram of my left breast. She recommended having a needle biopsy to find out what it was. Then after examining my breast and viewing my mammogram, the surgeon recommended waiting and having another mammogram in six months. Of course I was relieved and managed to put the matter out of my mind for the duration. So it would seem the dream was giving me good news. Actually, it was a combination of bad news and good news, which I would discover and understand more fully later.

GETTING THE RESULTS

On Tuesday afternoon, February 1, I arrived for my appointment at 3:15 p.m. After I was taken back to an examining room, I undressed from the waist up, slipped on the gown, and stretched out on the table to wait for the doctor's arrival. I heard him go into a room next to mine. After he finished there, I heard a nurse go into another room and announce that the doctor had been called back to the operating room. Soon she came in to me and gave me the same information. She said she could go ahead and take the stitches out and I could come back another day to see him. She thought he might be gone up to thirty minutes. We needed to get Owen to an appointment at the Richmond Health and Wellness Center at 5:00 p.m.

"My main concern is to get the report. It's okay for you to take out the stitches," I said. She looked in my folder and looked at the pathology report, then announced, "The doctor will have to tell you about the report." When she said this I knew something was wrong.

"Would you please go to the waiting room to tell Owen the doctor was delayed?" I asked. Several minutes later I decided I wanted Owen to come back to me, so I left the room, walked around the corner of the hall holding my gown closed, and asked another nurse to tell the first nurse to ask Owen to come back.

Before long he appeared and I told him what was going on. I

became most eager to get to see what the report said. I wanted to ask to be shown it right away, not waiting for the doctor to return. I noticed that my folder had been taken out of the "slot" on the door. The nurse must have feared we'd take it upon ourselves to look at it. She might have been right.

About that time we heard the doctor's voice as he was returning. He came into the room followed by a young intern and the nurse. We were introduced to the intern. "I tried to get you twice on Friday," Dr. Swensson announced.

I thought to myself, "You evidently didn't try all afternoon." We had gone out to lunch and I was home by 2:00 p.m.

"I got the answering machine and didn't want to leave any message on this. Then, too, I knew you would be coming in on Tuesday. It is cancer."

There. It'd been said. I was in a daze. I tried to listen as the doctor continued.

"I recommend either a lumpectomy or a mastectomy followed by radiation and maybe chemotherapy."

I was unable to take in much of what the doctor told us at that time. He said more, I'm sure, but I cannot remember. My reading since then tells me that women hearing the pronouncement of cancer usually hear no more than 10% of what the doctor says at this time. I know I didn't absorb much more. Owen was there, of course, and reported to me a little more that he remembered. Recently he told me that upon hearing the news he had a visceral reaction and felt slightly faint. He said he was glad he was sitting down.

Swensson asked me if I had any questions. "I'm sure I'll have some, but I don't know enough to ask more now," I replied. "I'd like to have copies of the pathology reports."

He suggested I might want to consult with a radiation therapist, a medical oncologist, and a reconstruction doctor (a plastic surgeon).

Rosa, his secretary who does the scheduling of appointments, wanted to know if I'd like to call from there to make other appointments.

"No," I said. "We'll wait and talk it over before doing so."

Rosa gave me the names and phone numbers of the various doctors suggested.

We managed to get away in time to get me to Willow Lawn Shopping Center before Owen was due at his appointment. He let me off at the mall, where I went to a nearby bookstore and spent the time looking through the books on cancer. I was determined to find out everything I could to fight the disease, to rid my body of the invading cells. I chose five books to buy: two giving medical information and three "inspirational" ones by people who have survived cancer.

I was in a daze, perhaps in shock, most of the way home. Neither Owen nor I can recall any conversation. I was experiencing a multitude of emotions—shock, disbelief, and fear. My inner being made silent protest with an unspoken cry of: "I'm not ready to depart this world. There's so much more I want to do, to contribute. I'm not ready to leave Owen. I expect to have thirty more years with him."

Recall now the dream of June 16 about microscopic organisms. After Dr. Swensson recommended waiting six months and having another mammogram, I assumed the dream had a positive message. It did. But it also pointed out a serious problem. The spot on the mammogram was cancer. The dream wasn't showing a plague of insects on a landscape, but I take the image of microscopic organisms crawling on my skin and entering a tiny opening to be a similar metaphor. Dreams come with messages from our unconscious, but we can't always understand right away what the message is. Sometimes other events need to take place and our knowledge of metaphors and symbols needs to build before we can understand. This becomes evident as my experience with cancer unfolds, as I try to be guided by dreams.

Looking back at this dream now I can see that the white substance which I squeezed out was a symbol for the cancer. Had I thought of this at the time, I certainly would have been very worried during the six-months wait. But if I had taken notice of the last several lines, I could have felt encouraged about my situation. The dream specifically said that after the cancer was out it was no longer a problem. The lines stated: *I am relieved to know what the strange place on the skin has been about and that it is nothing of consequence and that it is out . . . . I am relieved to know what is going on and it is not a further problem.*

Meanwhile I dealt with the crisis I faced in the way that came most naturally to me. I began reading the medical books as soon as we arrived home. I felt compelled to learn all I could as quickly as possible about everything involved, including terminology, possible causes, and treatments, to help me make an informed decision about what surgery to have. I read until 4:00 a.m. before I was able to put the books down and finally fall asleep.

I didn't sleep more than three or four hours. I don't remember whether I awoke on my own or was awakened by the phone. Either way, I answered the phone to find my gynecologist's nurse saying that the doctor wanted to speak to me.

"I have gotten the report from Swensson's office," the doctor announced. "I'm glad you have gotten a biopsy and have caught the cancer early. It is small and can be treated."

Then she said that this meant no more estrogen. I reminded her that I was already stopping this, that I had just one or two partial pills left in the tapering off process and that I would not take them.

She recommended Dr. Shelton Horsley, a surgical oncologist who at that time was director of the Breast Clinic at the Medical College of Virginia, for consultation. She informed me that Dr. Swensson had trained under Dr. Horsley.

By mid-morning I began making phone calls, telling friends and family what was happening and seeking further advice and support. My strongest and most immediate support came from my husband. For this I was and am most grateful.

When we were discussing my situation a day or two after receiving the diagnosis, I was quite conscious that Owen was trying to contain his own emotions. I told him I knew he had his own fears and I wanted him to express them, not to hold them back in an attempt to keep my spirits up. It is an honorable and compassionate trait to strive to protect a loved one by concealing one's own fears and concerns, but it can be unhealthy. Both people concerned need to be able to express their thoughts and fears openly with each other. I believed this honest and open communication was of utmost importance.

I had a strong sense that holding in my feelings would be detrimental to my body. I wanted to release as much as I could in order to free my body and mind to fight cancer.
— Neil A. Fiore,
The Road Back to Health

2

Seeking Counsel and Support

Selecting a medical team that we have a high level
of confidence in is perhaps our first responsibility
after diagnosis.
— Greg Anderson,
The Cancer Conqueror:
An Incredible Journey to Wellness

In the midst of this crisis I wondered where to find help. Obviously, further surgery and maybe other treatments were needed, but I didn't know which way to turn. I was trying to get some basic information from the books so I would have at least a little background knowledge to help me understand what was going on.

My brother and sister-in-law counseled me to seek expert advice to help me select the best surgeon I could find. This certainly was my intention. I began making phone calls. I tried to reach both Dr. McLanahan and Dr. Sylvest. Sandra's answering machine announced that she would be away until Sunday morning. I left a message for Dr. Sylvest to call me.

I next spoke with Williamsburg resident Joan Windsor, an intuitive counselor and author of several books, including *Dreams and Healing,* whom I first met at a workshop of the same title. An intuitive counselor is one who can acquire medical or psychological information by direct intuition rather than through more objective means of transmission. I had gotten to know her better at another workshop and in private consultation. After I explained my situation to her, she said that I was going to be okay and then gave me much advice. She recommended having a lumpectomy, not a mastectomy, eating organic foods entirely and drinking filtered water. She thought I had Sandra McLanahan to thank for the cancer not spreading in the six months from June to December. She expressed confidence that it would all be over within three or four months. I sensed she felt intuitively more than she was saying at the time. She wanted me to call again after the various consultations. She was not sure I would need radiation or chemotherapy, stating that there are other approaches. She was leery of the side effects of chemotherapy, including liver damage. I told her I was also leery of the side effects of radiation.

Late morning, Dr. Sylvest returned my call. I told him the diagnosis was a "0.6 cm. mucinous (colloid) carcinoma." He said, "There is good prognosis with this kind of cancer. You should make sure to nurture yourself. Get worries about other people's concerns out of your mind. Your cancer could have been the result of 'over-mothering' on your part. I will call for the slides of your biopsy and have them sent to me. After looking at them, I will call you back. It might be two or three days before I have the slides in hand." I was very grateful to have him view my slides and pleased to hear the positive prognosis. Since he had been pathologist at Johnston-Willis Hospital for many years, he was an excellent person from whom to get a second opinion. I wasn't too sure how to take his statement about "over-mothering." I didn't know just how to put aside worries about other people's concerns and I thought I already did things that would be considered nurturing myself.

I also called several additional professional people with whom I had had various meaningful connections. One is an art therapist and teacher of the MARI (Mandala Assessment Research Institute) System of using mandalas in diagnosis and counseling of clients. I had taken Level I training in Mandala Assessment with her in the spring of 1994 and planned to take Level II at the end of the month. She said she would ask a patient of hers who had breast cancer to recommend some inspirational books, would include me in their "circle of light," and wanted to be kept informed of my progress.

Another is a massage therapist and Reiki Master with whom I had taken Levels I and II of Reiki training. Reiki is a form of energy medicine utilizing a method of healing similar to what is known as "healing touch." She gave me various bits of dietary advice and said she would send me long distance Reiki and would include me in their Wednesday prayer circle.

CONSULTATIONS WITH A HOLISTIC PHYSICIAN

> True holistic medicine must take the final step—that of bringing conventional and alternative wisdom together in an integrated fashion.
>
> — Drs. Michael Greenwood & Pete Nunn, *Paradox & Dreaming: Medicine, Mythology & Transformation*

Friday, February 4, Dr. McLanahan called me from St. Johns Island to let me know she had received my message. After being told my situation she asked, "Is lumpectomy followed by radiation one of the options you have been given? I think this is the best way to go."

"I have read McDougall. He doesn't seem to like this option," I replied. (John A. McDougall, M.D., is an author and creator of a nationally recognized diet and exercise program for treating and preventing disease.)

"We can help you rebuild your immune system after radiation. You should ask Vernon Sylvest for recommendations for a surgeon," she responded.

"I have already discussed this with him and I have asked him to take a look at the biopsy slides."

"Good for you," she responded. "Another of my patients had a mastectomy six to eight years ago. She is doing fine now. She had used meditation tapes while having chemotherapy and had few side effects from the chemo. It would be a good idea to talk with people who have had surgery to find out what they think about their doctors. I will be back tomorrow evening and we can get together soon for further discussion."

Four days later, I went to an appointment with Dr. McLanahan, this time in Yogaville, forty miles northwest of our home. She gave me a magnetic treatment with her magnatherm machine for twenty to twenty-five minutes. I was puzzled about the procedure. She explained that this bolsters the immune system and helps in healing, thus helping prevent the spread of cancer. In a later conversation she gave a fuller explanation. "This machine sends out pulsations of a special kind of electromagnetic energy that allows the body to do better repair work. I gave you the treatment to help prepare you for the lumpectomy. The machine hasn't been proven enough to use it alone without other treatment."

She thought the cancer was related to taking estrogen, stress, and the loss of my father, who died in December of 1991. She said deep sadness can affect the immune system. She recommended watching a video entitled *Fight for Your Life,* which features Bernie Siegel and others. She said she had lost her copy, but thought Vernon Sylvest had one.

Dr. McLanahan gave diet recommendations which included no sugars, fruit juices or sweeteners; eating more raw food; and taking a lower dose of vitamin E (reduce from 800 mg. to 400 mg.). She also recommended Country Grown Cereal "Favorite Mixed Five Grains" and acidophilus, the kind that is grown on brown rice. She recommended getting the book *Prescription for Nutritional Healing* by James F. Balch and Phyllis A. Balch. As to special supplements, she recommended taking extra vitamin A, oil based 25,000 IU daily, extra echinacea, and arnica, a homeopathic remedy, at the time of surgery.

Some other suggestions included:

1. Before going to sleep at night I should ask for a dream for information, such as "What am I angry about?" (I wasn't aware I was or might be angry about anything and I had no idea why she thought this was related to getting cancer.)

2. After going to a quiet place in the car I should scream and yell to see what comes up.

3. She recommended seeing a holistic oncologist in Norfolk. She speculated that it would take six months to get in to see him, but thought it would be worth it to be advised by him.

4. She thought the best wisdom would be to use adjunctive therapies along with lumpectomy and radiation. I should ask for local anesthesia for the lumpectomy, which she considered a lot less toxic than a general anesthetic.

5. At first she said she didn't think tamoxifin was very effective. But then she said tamoxifin might be helpful for me with my situation, perhaps because my estrogen receptors were positive.

From a psychological perspective, she was of the opinion that I identify more with my masculine side because of my strong relation to my father. She said I "should allow Owen to give more. I should create space to allow it to happen."

She told me she was writing a medical book with her brother. She would photocopy the chapter on breast cancer to send to me. What I later received was part of the first draft of their book, *Surgery and Its Alternatives,* mentioned at the beginning of this book.

When I called her the next afternoon, I asked more questions. She had previously recommended our buying spring water to drink. "Should we get it in glass bottles?" I asked.

"Yes, glass is better [than plastic]," she replied.

"Should I have the lymph nodes taken out to see if they are cancerous?" I asked.

"It depends on whether the treatment you would agree upon would be different if we took them out and knew what they showed," she responded. "You need to discuss this with the people involved."

We discussed some of the remedies that she had prescribed the day before. Following this conversation I placed an order for various items.

> It is a rare physician indeed who searches beyond the symptoms of physical illnesses to find the impact of ideas and feelings on a patient's physical health.
>
> — Drs. Michael Greenwood & Pete Nunn,
> *Paradox & Dreaming:*
> *Medicine, Mythology & Transformation*

INFORMATION FROM FRIENDS

After the February 4 conversation with Sandra McLanahan, I followed her suggestion to get people's opinions about doctors. I called a friend at Hampden-Sydney who went through a mastectomy many years back. Her surgery had been performed by Dr. Horsley, whom my gynecologist had recommended. My friend thought he was great—businesslike, but very nice. She informed me that he is a busy doctor and might not be easy to get in to see, but that telling his secretary that it's a known cancer might make it easier to get to see him quickly. She praised him further, noting his kind interest, his taking time talking with her, but not wasting time. She had every confidence in him and said he would be on top of the situation. She wanted me to let her know when I would get to see him and then when the surgery was planned. She offered to go with me for follow-ups and help in any way.

I decided to try to get an appointment and called Dr. Horsley's office. I was told his secretary would call me back early Monday morning. They might be able to get me an appointment on the 10th, which was less than a week away.

Sunday afternoon I had extended conversations with two other acquaintances who had had hospital experiences. One's husband had been at the hospital in question. She reported that the doctors were great but students kept coming in and checking on everything. Then the doctors would come in for rounds with the students. The other person, a seventy-eight year old woman who had a radical mastectomy, reported her experience with a local doctor in Farmville. She had liked him and had thought he had done a good job. She reported that her surgery had "not been pleasant to face," but she was glad that she had had it done when she did. She had decided against chemotherapy and was taking tamoxifin.

One friend, a nurse, advised doing something further, such as a lumpectomy. She thought it would be unwise to do nothing more. She said she knows that "we" (meaning patients) would like someone to tell us what to do, but the doctors would leave it up to me to decide what should be done. I told her I knew I needed to be the one to decide. I did have concerns about the possible side effects of the common methods of treatment. Only by weighing in my mind as much information as possible might I come to decisions I would feel were right for me. I knew from my prior reading what Bernie Siegel would later state in the preface of *Surgery and Its Alternatives*: "Studies have indicated that those who know their options and make their own choices are likely to do better." My friend further advised me to listen to whomever I had confidence in. I had told her that I had talked with Sandra McLanahan and that she recommended the lumpectomy and radiation. She said she knew I had confidence in Sandra.

Another professional whose opinion I valued was Dr. Tony Munoz, a local surgeon. He is also a family friend and former watercolor student of mine. I called him to ask about Dr. Horsley. He assured me that Horsley was "one of the best." During this call and a later one he said for me to tell Dr. Horsley that I was his friend. He thought the personal connection might be helpful. He declared my "chances of full recovery" were very good and he wished me "good luck."

On Monday, February 7, when I secured an appointment with Dr. Horsley for the following Thursday, his secretary wanted to know if the appointment was for a second opinion or to have the surgery done. I replied I wouldn't know for sure until I had seen the doctor, but I was leaning strongly towards having him do it.

When I spoke with Rosa at Dr. Swensson"s office later, she told me they had received the estrogen receptor report. The reading was: 80 staining positive to estrogen, 60 staining positive to progesterone. I took mental note of this. Recalling some information I had read, I decided this should mean I would be a candidate for taking tamoxifin, if needed.

CONVERSATION WITH A PATHOLOGIST AND HOLISTIC PHYSICIAN

During a phone conversation Tuesday morning Dr. Sylvest announced, "The prognosis is good. The cancer is not likely to be in the lymph nodes. I think Swensson is a good surgeon. You should see a radiologist if you see this as a part of the therapy you agree upon. It really doesn't matter what you do on a physical level. In this case a lumpectomy and radiation is a reasonable approach. I'm not even sure radiation is needed on this lesion." He repeated, "The prognosis is good on this kind of tumor and the suggestion of a lumpectomy with possible radiation is good. An alternative would be mastectomy. But I have never seen your particular kind of cancer having any lymph node involvement."

Elaborating on the comment that it really didn't matter what I do on a physical level, he said, "You need to focus on being relaxed and less concerned on making everyone around you happy. You need to reduce stress and your need to 'over-mother.' Then whatever you will do will work. You need to focus on being relaxed, on joy, on love, on gratitude every moment. All molecules will live blissfully. It takes discipline of the mind."

"Do you think it wise to have surgery?" I asked him again.

"I recommend a lumpectomy," he replied. "I think the physicians may say to have radiation following surgery. You should do what is most comfortable for you."

"What might be the side effects of radiation?" I asked.

"If you focus on it with love and trust, you shouldn't have any problems," he replied. "The side effects listed in books are those which come to those who don't have the above approach. Radiation is localized to the breast. They probably got all the cancer on the initial biopsy. But I assume they want to go back to take out a little more tissue."

He said he would send the slides directly to Dr. Horsley, so they will be there for my appointment.

I took time to inquire about his activities. One morning, one evening, and Saturdays he was counseling at the Richmond Health and Wellness Center. Progress on his book was coming along nicely. His book, *The Formula,* was published in 1997.

"Owen and I appreciate all you have done and all that has led to where we are now."

"It is very healing to hear this," he responded.

"I wish I had known what I know now years ago," I added.

"You weren't ready for it then. But the past doesn't exist. What is important is now," he assured me.

"Yes, we had discussed the idea that it took my going through what I have to get to the point where I am now." I also asked, "Have you seen the report from the estrogen receptor test?"

"Yes, I have and it was good."

I felt grateful to Dr. Sylvest for viewing the slides and reassured to hear such a positive prognosis. Despite this, I still was uneasy about what might be ahead for me. I wasn't convinced as to what measures I needed to take. If surgery was indeed needed, I wanted to find the best surgeon. Should I ask Dr. Horsley? He certainly was highly recommended by other doctors, nurses, and patients. I needed to continue seeking answers to questions spoken and unspoken.

I was glad I was encouraged to take my time to consider the next step—to decide what surgery to have performed, what surgeon to do it, and when. As I heard during conversations with others, some women proceed to have their surgery within a few days of learning their diagnosis, feeling it urgent to have it done as quickly as possible. I understood that my particular cancer was a "slow-moving" kind; additional days—and as it turned out, a few additional weeks—wouldn't make any difference. I was very thankful for that. I wanted to investigate my options as carefully as possible. I was fortunate to have doctors who did not "push"; they assured me the choice of what treatments and how much or how little was mine to make.

> What you choose to believe about cancer is crucial to your journey. . . . Your beliefs about the disease, the treatment, and your role have incredible power over the outcome. You can choose those beliefs.
>
> — Greg Anderson,
> *The Cancer Conqueror: An Incredible Journey to Wellness*

SHARING THE NEWS

The day after I received the diagnosis of breast cancer I began making many phone calls—some to family and friends letting them know what was happening and asking for their prayers and support. The news began to spread. Wednesday afternoon, a week after my initial diagnosis, I saw two friends while down town. One said she didn't know if she was supposed to know about my illness. I told her I didn't mind. We had a lengthy discussion and she expressed concern and sympathy and said she'd keep checking on me.

My feelings were and continue to be that it is good to let people know what is going on. I certainly didn't feel I should hide my problem. Having breast cancer is not shameful, but this was a prevalent feeling years ago that still lingers with some people. For many years the word cancer has brought fear to the hearts and minds of almost everyone. Some doctors would not even tell their patient he/she had cancer. The diagnosis would be discussed with family members who would then keep it a secret from their loved ones. Those who knew of the illness would not speak its name, certainly not to other people. Fortunately times are changing, at least for some.

I also hoped by discussing my situation I might help others.

One friend admitted she hadn't gone for either a mammogram or a gynecological exam in eight years. She said she disliked these exams so much she kept putting them off. Knowing that early detection can be life saving, I urged her to go.

The second person I saw that day in February worked at a department store and greeted me warmly, asking how I was (not knowing about the cancer). I said I was great in some ways, but I had a problem. Then I told her what had been going on. She asked where I would have surgery. When I said probably MCV (since, at that time, I was seriously considering having Dr. Horsley as the surgeon), she praised the hospital profusely. Her husband had been there during his last illness. She said the doctors, staff, and everyone were very good and very kind. I told her that made me feel good to know this.

Later that day another friend called and wanted to come right over. We discussed various aspects of the cancer. I told her about my "initial dreams" and let her read the one about the two men. As she left, she was fighting back tears and declared I was an inspiration.

Another person said she already knew about my cancer, but she didn't know if we were telling other people. She appreciated being told and talking about it. After seeking advice from various doctors and professionals, I made calls to many friends, some had been my roommates and close friends as far back as prep school and college. I wanted their prayers, their healing vibrations of love which I felt would be sent my way. Some people recounted tales of friends and relatives who had had cancer. Most gave positive accounts. Occasionally someone, without thinking of the possible effect it might have, would tell of a friend or relative who had died of breast cancer. But this did not upset me. I guess it might have had I been having a bad time or if my prognosis were not good. I listened with great interest and empathy as others told me about their own experiences with cancer.

One acquaintance—at the end of our conversation—said she wanted me to keep her "abreast" of what was going on. Immediately she said, "Whoops! That wasn't the right thing to say." "That's okay," I replied. "I'm not sensitive to that type of comment." That kind of slip of the tongue just added a bit of humor to the conversation.

3

Taking Note of Dreams

By tapping into dreams, we come into contact with
the intelligence that is creating our lives.
— Angela Passidomo Trafford,
The Heroic Path: One Woman's Journey from Cancer to Self-Healing

For several years I had been keeping a dream journal, writing down whatever dream or dream fragments I remembered first thing in the morning. I began an informal program of study of the meaning of dreams, reading some of the few books on the subject I could find at the time and attending a brief weekend seminar led by Joan Windsor. I marveled at the idea that the meaning of dreams could be deciphered.

After I learned on Tuesday, February 1, that I had breast cancer, I decided I should take note of any dreams I had, to see what they might tell me about my situation. I remembered a series of six dreams, which I will subsequently refer to as the "initial dream series," when I woke on Friday morning. I am attending some kind of educational conference in the dreams and the various "scenes" are somehow connected.

I Fear the Woman is Drowning

1. I am in a crowd of people in "grandstand" seats at the edge of water. I am on the first row, right beside the water. I see a woman either jump in or fall in. I am alarmed and fearful for her. I think someone needs to jump in and rescue her. I am afraid she will drown. I look around to see if anyone is going to do anything to help. No one seems to be making a move. I watch as she goes under and doesn't come back up. Since nobody is jumping in, I feel I need to, even though I am fully clothed. I am not sure how well I can help. Before I do jump, I see her finally resurface a slight distance away, coming up beyond some people or other obstacles a few feet farther away. She may "sputter" a little, but she doesn't seem to need more help.

The Short Man Easily and Gently Carries Me

2. I am with two men. One is thin and shorter than the other. He looks at me very kindly and somehow I know he wants to pick me up and carry me. I say I think I am much too big and heavy for him. The other man is bigger, taller. He is just standing there doing and saying nothing. I don't know the men; I don't know their names. The shorter man responds that he can lift me: "We'll see what I can do." He very slowly and gently eases me up so I am horizontal and am being held close to him. I wonder somewhat at his doing this, whether it is okay since I am married. But it feels okay and right and I feel safe and secure. He doesn't try to lift me high, just so I am maybe at his waist or chest level. He then slowly and gently eases and turns me around, moving me several feet farther over in the room or space where we are. It may be more a hallway than a room. I think I am amazed at the ease and gentleness with which he does this.

I Choose to Stay In and Rest

3. There are various happenings and details related to the meeting (conference) that I don't now remember. One may have to do with meals. One has to do with some people in the group making plans for recreation one evening: to go out and away from the conference place one evening. I think I say I'll just stay there and rest.

I Go into the Men's Room

4. At one point I need the bathroom. I find one and go in. While in there I realize I have gone in the men's room. I don't want to be found in there and I don't want anyone to know I have gone in the wrong place. I don't think anyone knows or realizes what has happened.

I Dump the Excrement into a Man's Cap

5. I am carrying a container that has excrement in it. I'm not sure whether it is mine or somehow I have collected or picked up some. Anyhow, I am looking around (outside on open ground) for a place to get rid of it. I see something that looks like a small container on the ground, so I dump the stuff in there. I am surprised to see some man come along looking around on the ground. He seems to touch this object with his lip or mouth as if testing to see if it is what he is looking for. The idea of his doing this repulses me. I certainly think this is strange. He then picks it up and I am either told or realize somehow that the container is his cap. I am very alarmed that I had dumped the shit into it. I think I am apologetic and try to explain what I had done, not realizing the container was a hat. The man doesn't seem concerned. A crowd of people who are around and have seen what is happening actually laugh and/or snicker at the whole incident.

The Man Wants Me to Participate in His Group

6. There is a group of people who have participated in the conference and who have been with a particular man in a small discussion group. The man is arranging seats and is either putting name signs on the seats or making a list of people to take part in a future session with him. He sees me and wants to, and, I think, goes ahead and includes me in his group. It seems he wants me to be a part of it. He seems to be choosing people he thinks will be interested and good contributors to the discussions and sessions.

This sequence of dreams covers a wide variety of activities. I certainly didn't know how to interpret them in their entirety right away. I did think the first dream was illustrating my precarious situation and my reaction to it. I felt I was the woman the "I" in the dream—the ego—feared was drowning and I thought I needed to do something to save myself. Blinded by my initial anxiety over my diagnosis, I failed to see the positive outcome in this dream: she comes up from under the water on her own power. Although she may sputter, she doesn't seem to need more help.

I believed the second dream in the series was very significant for the present time; it might help answer the question uppermost in my mind: Who should perform the lumpectomy? I had an appointment to see Dr. Shelton Horsley at MCV for a second opinion. I also thought I might want him to do the lumpectomy. When my friend was telling me about Dr. Horsley, she described him as being small in stature and slim with white hair. I wondered if he fit what I sensed intuitively about the helping man in the second dream. Thinking this dream might be telling me who should be my surgeon, I began to give serious consideration to the description of the doctors.

I will discuss the various dreams as each became more clearly understood. I do believe the "initial dream series" was of pivotal importance, providing an overview of my entire experience with cancer. I've already mentioned what I saw as the significance of the first two dreams. As it has turned out, the other four pointed to means of healing and showed future events. At the time I could see only what the dreams were saying on an external, and at times literal, level. My mind was so caught up with the immediate medical experience and my working knowledge of dream symbolism was so limited that I missed the deeper, inner symbolism. I forgot that all characters in a dream can be symbols for parts of myself. Thus, the various men in this series of dreams can represent inner "animus" figures, parts of myself that have what we consider "masculine" attributes and were available to help me through this experience. I relate in this chapter how the second dream figured into my consideration of who should perform the lumpectomy.

> I've dreamt in my life dreams that have stayed with me ever after, and changed my ideas; they've gone through and through me, like wine through water, and altered the color of my mind.
>
> —Emily Brontë

THE APPOINTMENT WITH A SURGEON

Wednesday morning Dr. Horsley's office called and changed my appointment to the following day. Again we worried about the weather report which forecast rain and freezing rain for the next day.

Early Thursday morning we called Dr. Horsley's office to postpone the appointment. The threat of freezing rain and sleet appeared to be materializing. We had to settle on the following Thursday. We could call again on Monday to see if there was any chance of getting an appointment for Tuesday due to a cancellation.

I became very upset and angry at having to postpone the appointment. The more I thought about it, the more the anger festered inside me. Later, when I was alone in the house and thus wouldn't upset Owen with my behavior, I let it all out, crying tears of release, screaming and yelling at the top of my lungs. I certainly understood the need for caution due to the weather, but I didn't like to have to wait another week to see Horsley. If the secretary had said we could have an appointment Monday or Tuesday it wouldn't have upset me so much. I was surprised at the fierceness of the anger. As I reflect upon the incident, I sense it wasn't just about the immediate postponement. It may have been more a release of unconscious and unexpressed anger at having cancer. Allowing myself to express the built-up tension and anger could be healing. Come to think of it, this was what Sandra McLanahan had in mind. She obviously was aware of the studies that show that cancer patients who express their feelings get along better than those who do not.

I called Dr. Swensson's office to let Rosa know we would not be picking up the mammogram films because of the weather conditions. She said a week's postponement to the following Thursday wouldn't make any difference.

That evening, our son Russ called from his home in Chattanooga, Tennessee. Thinking I had seen Dr. Horsley that day, he was calling to find out what we had learned. We told him of our disappointment in having to postpone this meeting a week.

Friday evening, my brother Russell called from Columbia, Maryland and suggested we call our cousin who is a retired surgeon to get his input. Russell also assured us we'd be welcome at their house if we should want to consult at Johns Hopkins. I appreciated his interest and concern.

The ice storm did indeed materialize. We lost electricity, ate a cold meal of vegetable salad and cereal, and sat near a kerosene heater listening to a Bernie Siegel tape until going to bed early. Saturday morning we discovered that one of our large willow trees in the front yard was demolished—brittle limbs and the trunk broken by the weight of ice.

When we finally saw Dr. Horsley he announced that the biopsy slides had arrived earlier (days ago probably), but he had not looked at them yet because he didn't know "what was up." I asked about the estrogen receptor test results. "It showed slightly positive," he informed us. "The cancer was small and the prognosis is good. Did you take Premarin?"

"I had, but I just recently stopped," I replied.

"Premarin would not have given you the cancer," he said, sensing my concern.

"One doctor thought it might have contributed," I responded.

"I'd like to be shown the proof," he retorted. He went on to suggest that I get another mammogram on the right breast "just to be sure that everything is all right since it was last done in June of '93 and you've lost a lot of weight since then. I don't have any reason to believe there is more cancer, but I will write to Dr. Swensson recommending this. I think you're in a very good set-up with the pathology report and what I see on the mammogram and the physical exam."

We expressed an interest in having him perform the surgery. "I couldn't do the surgery for three weeks," he replied. "No, I'm right up to my eyeballs. I can tell you Erik will do a very good job. I just can't do it. I appreciate your interest."

"If Swensson does the surgery who will do the follow up with the oncologist?" Owen asked. "Do we come back here?"

"No, whoever is the surgeon should do the follow up," Dr. Horsley replied.

"In other words, she doesn't need an additional oncologist?" Owen questioned again.

"No, not unless she has positive nodes or something of that nature that she would want to get treated. There is a handsome group of oncologists out there—a whole group of oncologists out there. They are graduates of here. I'll leave it up to his [Swensson's] discretion. The way we work it here, I follow my patients that I operate on. I see them every six months. Dr. Belgrad or someone on his staff will follow you."

"Where is he?" I asked.

"Johnston-Willis," he replied. "He was here a couple years ago, and did a very good job. I think you're a good candidate. I don't think there's any problem."

Dr. Horsley then elaborated on the approach he would follow if he were doing it. He would not do a further lumpectomy at the biopsy site. But he would do the axillary excision of lymph nodes, which would entail a separate incision from the lumpectomy.

When I told him that Dr. Swensson recommended a further lumpectomy, he looked at the pathology report again and said, "Swensson might think it best to take more (breast tissue) to be sure. I would give the area a "boost" in radiation, instead of further surgery."

I asked about the notion of rotating breast tissue to close the gap in the breast, as one of the books I had read mentioned. He said this is not a good idea. "It is better to leave breast tissue in its normal place. I don't think you need any further tests such as a bone scan. The lumpectomy is equally as good as the mastectomy for you, and it does save the breast." He explained that radiation is done for five days a week for six weeks and recommended having it done at Johnston-Willis.

I asked if the tenderness at the biopsy site three weeks after it was done is normal.

"Yes, it is."

I asked how long the hospital stay would be (I think I said for a lumpectomy).

"Three or four days," he said. "Joanne" at Swensson's office had told me that at Johnston-Willis a lumpectomy stay is usually twenty-three hours. You go in the morning of the operation and stay one night.

When I asked Dr. Horsley whether lumpectomy is done with anesthesia or a local, he wanted to know what doctor suggested "local" for it. I didn't tell him. He recommended using anesthesia.

I had gone to my appointment with Dr. Horsley eager to see

if he seemed to fit the description of the shorter man in the second dream of February 4. I wondered if he should be my surgeon. Dr. Horsley was relatively shorter than Dr. Swensson and was kind, but I didn't get the feeling that he was the man. He had also ruled himself out as surgeon by stating that he was "up to his eyeballs for the next three weeks" and I should go ahead and have Dr. Swensson do the surgery.

After leaving Horsley's office we went to Swensson's office, thinking I would return the mammograms there. They wanted me to keep them to deliver to later appointments, which Joanne helped make. One was for the mammogram of the right breast for the next day at Chippenham Hospital, so we would have results before the appointment with Swensson on Friday. After checking Swensson's operating schedule she said he might be able to do the surgery on Wednesday of next week at Johnston-Willis Hospital.

The next morning I called Swensson's office to ask several questions. I learned that a nurse at the hospital would notify our insurance company. I would have to call later to learn the time of my operation. When I asked who made arrangements for admittance, she replied, "For a lumpectomy Swensson calls it 'a twenty-three hour outpatient procedure,' therefore, you will not be 'technically' admitted to the hospital. If the need should arise after the operation for you to stay longer, you will then be 'admitted' to the hospital. But not for more than a total of forty-eight hours, unless you develop complications. This is what the insurance company requires. It is the 'doctor's call' on what the length of stay is. With the twenty-three hour deal the stay is for observation and it cannot be in a private room."

"Dr. Horsley indicated the stay would be three or four days," I told her.

"This would be for a mastectomy."

"We only discussed the lumpectomy. Would it be one way at one hospital and another at the other," I asked.

"It is the doctor who decides what his policy is for what type of operation, " she responded.

That afternoon I went to Woman's Clinic at Chippenham Hospital to get the mammogram. There I found that I had not been put on the schedule, even though Joanne had called and arranged it the afternoon before. They called "scheduling" and found they had no record of the appointment. After I explained what was going on, why I was to have the mammogram, they said they would go ahead and do it. After the procedure was completed the nurse said that Dr. Swensson didn't usually want them to give the results to the patient, but she wanted to and would in this case. The mammogram on the right breast showed no change since June. She wished me well.

ADVICE FROM A SURGEON FRIEND

At this point I was still trying to decide what to do. Hoping to get some further insights I called Dr. Tony Munoz and explained that Horsley could not do the surgery. He assured me that Swensson is a very good surgeon. "You will be in very good hands. Although Swensson doesn't have as much experience as Horsley, I wouldn't hesitate to have him for Mary Ellen [Tony's wife]. I would be looking for experience when choosing Horsley."

"How does Johnston-Willis Hospital compare to Chippenham?" I asked.

"The same group of doctors work at them and the facilities are equal," he replied. " They are as good as other hospitals such as St. Mary's and Henrico." When told Horsley's opinion to not take more out at the site, Tony said he agreed. "Less taken out would be my preference. Yes, I do think lymph nodes should be taken out, so you can know better the prognosis. No nodes positive would be excellent. If this is the case I will be all smiles. One to five nodes positive is very good. Over five nodes the chances diminish."

"What is the difference between sampling and dissection?" I asked.

"Sampling means they take out several nodes. In a dissection they take all the nodes. The operation on the nodes, even the dissection, is not a 'big' operation in the surgeon's eyes. The axillary node operation is not big. But I know that any operation is 'big' for the patient. As to the length of stay in the hospital, it is just twenty-three hours for the sampling and this is not really a problem. The stay with a dissection would be longer because it is a more involved operation."

"What is the potential of cutting nerves during the axillary operation?"

"I have never done so myself and have not heard of anyone else doing so, although I have read of it and know it is a concern," he replied.

"What do you think about using only a local anesthetic?"

"I would not advise having the axillary operation under local anesthetic."

"Do we need to consult a medical oncologist now before the surgery?"

"Not now, afterwards, if Swensson wants this done. Swensson will arrange for this and/or with a radiotherapist probably, depending upon his usual procedures. I used to do the follow up myself because there wasn't an oncologist coming to Farmville. Please keep me posted. I'm still your friend."

I appreciated the input from Tony, and his good wishes. Next I tried to check back in with several people with whom I had consulted earlier. I got Joan Windsor's answering machine. Vernon Sylvest was in Seattle, Washington, and would be back the following Monday. Sandra McLanahan wouldn't be back in Richmond until March 2. She went to Washington, D.C., the day before, to give a speech.

ADVICE FROM AN INTUITIVE COUNSELOR

After supper Joan Windsor returned my call. She wished I would have a better surgeon. "I think you should wait. You would be better off with Horsley. It sounds as if you aren't satisfied with Swensson."

"I liked him okay in June when we first consulted him," I said. "But he wasn't good at communication. Both Vernon and Tony say Swensson is a good surgeon. But he doesn't have the experience that Horsley has."

"I wonder if Horsley might get a cancellation and be able to take you before three weeks. What did Vernon have to say?"

"I haven't reported back to him yet."

"Wait 'till Vernon comes back," she advised. "I think he will probably have the answer. Will waiting two more weeks be a problem? If Vernon thinks it won't hurt to wait, that will be the answer."

"I think he probably will think it all right to wait since he thinks that all the cancer has been gotten out at the biopsy."

I also told her about the differing recommendations regarding the surgery between Horsley and Swensson and that Tony Munoz had agreed with Horsley. Also there seemed to be a difference in the length of stay in the hospital, if I was correct in remembering Horsley said it would be three or four days for a lumpectomy.

I told her my dream about the two men. She thought the dream was saying who should do the surgery and it was Horsley. She urged me not to commit to anything the next day and suggested I could make a tentative schedule and then maybe could cancel.

"I'm not as favorably inclined towards MCV for the hospital (where Horsley would be) as Johnston-Willis (where Swensson would operate)," I added. "I'm very confused at this point."

Joan Windsor takes into consideration numerology and astrology when making decisions. "I think it would be better to wait. But I hate to tell you to wait, in case I'm wrong. Wednesday is not a good day. Even if you choose Swensson for the surgeon I don't think Wednesday is a good day for the surgery."

Checking the calendar she noted the full moon would be Friday, the 26th of February. "Don't do anything on the full moon," she advised further. "Call me back at 10:00 p.m. I will get my astrologer friend to pick a better date. According to astrology, now is a time when communications are difficult. Nothing may be as it seems. One thing is said to you and it turns out differently."

When I called Joan back, she announced that her friend didn't feel any urgent need for quick surgery. She then proceeded to tell me to avoid certain dates and stated which dates would be good. She went on to explain that things go well on the waning moon. Various parts of the body are ruled by different astrological signs, the breast by the sign Cancer. So when the moon goes through the sign of Cancer, don't operate on the breast. This was to be happening the following week. She said signs change every two and one-half days and on unfavorable days things might not go as well. You might have bleeding or other complications. But the long range prognosis would not be affected. She told me that when her husband, mother, and mother-in-law all had surgery they had carefully picked dates and they all did really well. She said this would give me some dates to consider, but that I had to make the decision as to which surgeon and which date.

After the phone call I was exceedingly confused. How much weight should I give to Joan's advice? I had read elsewhere (in fact, Sandra McLanahan stated in her book, parts of which I had just read in manuscript form) that it is not good to have an operation at the full moon because there might be more bleeding. I believe there is something to this. I didn't know what to think about the numerology and astrology.

Joan does believe in the importance of dreams, as I do. I was so excited right after the dream about the two men. After talking with my friend about Dr. Horsley I thought he might be the one who should be the surgeon. But, I told Joan, I wondered if this were correct or if there were someone else out there that should do it. I didn't feel that Dr. Horsley's appearance exactly fit the feeling I had about the short, slim man in the dream.

The next morning, Friday, I awoke remembering the following dream.

The Man Avoids Me; My Friend Goes On Ahead of Me

I'm on a street of a city or town and I'm waiting, hoping a man I'm interested in will be walking up my way so I would meet up with him. I am romantically interested in him. But I have a feeling he might not be interested in me. I look around the corner and down the sidewalk by the buildings to see if he is coming. I spot him coming up the sidewalk, which may be slightly uphill, in my direction. I hastily go back around the corner so he won't see me. I want it to look as if we are casually and accidentally meeting as he reaches the corner. I wait, but he does not appear in a few minutes. I figure he may have spotted me and decided to go in a different direction to avoid me. I hang around a little while. A female friend of mine comes by and I start walking along with her, chatting. I ask her about her social life, if she is having any dates. She says she has had a few. I reply that is at least better than I have done, that I am not having any these days. I am pleased that I am walking along with her. I'm enjoying her companionship. But soon she goes on ahead of me around

> *the edge of a pond or pool that has rocks at the point. She climbs up onto a rock that projects over the water and begins reading a newspaper, or something similar, that she is holding. I feel deserted and left on my own.*

After studying the dream I came up with a possible interpretation: Maybe the man I'm interested in is the surgeon I'm looking for and hope will have some interest in me. That could be Dr. Horsley. (In dream interpretation you don't have to take dream facts literally, therefore the "interest" doesn't have to be romantic.) "Going in a different direction" is his not wanting to do my surgery at this time. Perhaps the female friend was Joan Windsor, who has "dates"—when I should have the operation. (Dreams can use different meanings of words to make the point.) My not having any dates might correspond to the fact that the date for my operation has not yet been set. The friend going on ahead and leaving me alone might represent my having to make my own decisions.

Then I had a new insight into a possible meaning of the "two men" dream. It crossed my mind that perhaps the dream was referring not to a choice between surgeons, but was showing who would help following the surgery. The reference to the taller man "standing there doing and saying nothing" could mean that Dr. Swensson had completed his part and the shorter man was showing that he could help in a safe and gentle manner after the surgery. He might be the radiotherapist or oncologist rather the surgeon. I planned to ask Swensson or his secretary for a description of these men.

QUESTIONS ARE ANSWERED

> I insisted they share all information with me in terms I could understand. And I wanted explanations for each and every test. I had to be part of every treatment decision.
>
> — Greg Anderson,
> *The Cancer Conqueror:*
> *An Incredible Journey to Wellness*

In preparation for my appointment with Dr. Swensson, I made a four page list in longhand of questions to ask him and left spaces to write his answers. I felt that if he could give me satisfactory answers to these questions I would feel more comfortable with having him perform the lumpectomy. I found Swensson to be relaxed and open to questions. He seemed to realize I was informed and wanted detailed answers to the questions, so he patiently gave me answers, pausing to give me time to record them. He used medical terms with which I was familiar as a result of all the reading I had been doing.

I asked how much more tissue would be removed at the tumor site and how many nodes would be removed. He replied he intended to take 1 cm. around the site and including the site. He stated which nodes he would remove along with an axillary vein, two muscles, two intercostal nerves. He also explained the use of a drainage tube, what kind and how much radiation would be used later in treatment, and under what circumstances I might need chemotherapy.

I asked if there had been any excessive bleeding during the biopsy. I had the feeling that it took longer to finish than he first thought it might take. He replied the procedure went as it normally should. He was extracting loose breast tissue. Any oozing needed to be stopped so the area could be left absolutely dry.

After telling him I wanted to avoid any nausea such as I had after knee surgery, I asked if I should give him or some other person the information (which I had in my records) of what was used before. He replied I should give the anesthesiologist the information. The anesthesiologist would do whatever possible to avoid the nausea and usually could give something that wouldn't cause trouble.

I asked if it would be okay for me to listen to tapes with earphones during the surgery. I was thinking of making tapes of affirmations to listen to during the operation. He replied he preferred not to have extra wires in the OR. He said I'd be unconscious and wouldn't hear the tapes. His reply showed his main concern was unwanted wires since I know that an anesthetized person can be aware, at least in a subconscious way, of things said in one's presence. Bernie Siegel suggests telling your surgeon things to be said to you while under anthesthesia and for him or her to ask the staff to avoid making any negative remarks. He tells of getting positive results when he has asked patients, while they were under anesthesia, to help change their blood flow and blood pressure. Experience has shown him his patients can hear while anesthetized.

Dr. Swensson said for me to work out with his secretary arrangements for a private room and the date of the surgery. She could also tell me how to find the name of someone who has had a lumpectomy with and/or without radiation who would be willing to talk with me.

The complete list of my questions as I wrote them with the answers Dr. Swensson gave may be found in the Appendix.

Further discussion stated that radiation would begin a week or two after the staples are taken out from the surgery and will continue five weeks, five days a week.

I was pleased with this session with Swensson. Any feelings of a communication gap were dispelled. He listened to and answered questions in a very warm, caring manner. I felt much more at ease with the idea of his performing the lumpectomy. I let his secretary arrange an appointment for the radiation therapist the next week.

Rosa told me how good the woman radiologist was; she knew I would like her. I asked her to describe the man. She didn't know him, but she would ask the person she called to set up the appointment. This person described him as being "thin, short, balding with salt and pepper mustache." Thinking I would prefer the woman, Rosa was about to set up the appointment with her. But I announced that for personal reasons I wanted to have the appointment with the man. I did not tell her the reason, which was to see if he fit description and the "feel"—the compassion, consideration, concern—of the short man in my dream. I hoped she didn't think I'm prejudiced against female doctors. I definitely am not. I really appreciate the expertise and concern of my female gynecologist and all that Sandra McLanahan has done for me.

Rosa and the nurse were very interested to hear about what I'd been doing under Sandra McLanahan's guidance. The nurse got McLanahan's name and phone number from me and indicated she herself might want to consult her. They were also interested in how I was writing down all the information and went out of their way to provide detailed information on the pre-admission testing, which will include chest X-ray, medical history, a physical exam, EKG, and a variety of blood tests. I will be expected to bring my mammogram films with me for Dr. Belgrad.

MEETING WITH A RADIATION ONCOLOGIST

With great anticipation I went to my appointment the following Thursday with Dr. Richard Belgrad, radiation oncologist at Johnston-Willis Hospital. Owen went with me, as he did for each of the consultations. I wanted him to help me remember the information being given and to give me his opinions.

Oncology nurse "Marie" met with us first. She told us there would be thirty treatments.

"What are the potential side effects?" I asked.

"After ten to fifteen treatments you might have a feeling like a lump in the throat. For this we might prescribe Mylanta to be taken fifteen minutes before a meal or Carafate to soothe the esophagus, if the esophagus gets any of the radiation. There will be fatigue, but I think you could drive yourself to the treatments. With your fair skin, there might be 'pinking' of the skin. On Mondays we set aside extra time for the patient to talk with the doctor and nurses. On Tuesdays we do blood work every other week."

"Tell me about the simulation," I prompted.

"The simulation is done at the first session. It will take an hour. This will not be done until ten to fourteen days after surgery, waiting for the patient to gain motion in the arm, which has to be up over head for one hour during the simulation. We place a tattoo on the chest and/or breast to help line up exact placement for the treatments. Then the patient talks with Dr. Belgrad. Treatments will start a day or two later. We are off on national holidays. We also skip a day or two if the skin gets too pink or becomes raw. Then an aloe cream would be used."

"Dr. Belgrad is personable and takes a lot of time with his patients," Marie told us. "He'll take all the time you need. You might be interested to know that his son-in-law went to Hampden-Sydney."

Dr. Belgrad greeted us warmly when he came in. He took a long time getting to know us, making us feel at ease, even telling us about his family—in particular his sons, since both are artistic. Finally getting around to the medical matter at hand, he described the same potential side effects that the nurse did.

"Marie mentioned that there might be irritation of the esophagus. What about that?"

"I don't think the esophagus would be involved," he replied. "I would not treat any other areas, such as lymph nodes, under the breast, or the collar bone."

Regarding my particular treatment he explained, "I recommend treatments for five weeks with an additional week for the boost to the tumor bed. I would give a total of 6,000 units to the tumor bed and 4,500 units to the rest of the breast, given in approximately 180 units daily. We use two linear accelerators."

Dr. Belgrad had not seen the pathology slides yet. He thought Vernon Sylvest still had them. I told him I knew that Dr. Horsley had them after Dr. Sylvest saw them. Belgrad had taken thirty to forty minutes looking over the mammogram and other reports before coming in to see us. "You have an 'exceptionally favorable' situation," he announced. "There is a 'favorable connotation.' The cancer is 'extremely indolent.' It is very small, only .6 cm."

He recommended having the left breast mammogrammed again before surgery. I'm not sure why. He thought, as did Vernon Sylvest, that the cancer was gone. He did not think that the lymph nodes are involved; nor did he think I would need any chemotherapy or tamoxifin.

"Vernon Sylvest thinks I will be all right even if I do nothing further," I announced.

"Yes, I'm familiar with Vernon's approach to medicine. He is a good friend of mine." Upon reflection, Belgrad added, "Vernon might be right, but I believe for different reasons than does Vernon. But I think it a good idea to use a little radiation to eradicate any existing abnormalities."

"What do you think regarding estrogen possibly causing cancer?"

"The estrogen, given to you for years in HRT, may have stimulated some normal glandular changes that might have masked the situation. It might have been seen sooner otherwise, but this won't make any difference. There is no evidence that estrogen causes breast cancer."

"Should we consult with a medical oncologist at this point?"

"I don't think you need this. I don't think you have node involvement."

"Well then, do I even need the lumpectomy?" I asked. "Do I need to have further tissue taken?"

"I believe it is a good thing to do, since the margin was only .15 cm."

"I'm worried about the axillary dissection and the possible risks here. So I'd like not to have that done. If it were your wife, what would be your recommendation and preference?"

"That's a good question. I would probably opt for the taking of further breast tissue but pass on the axillary dissection. The chance of node involvement is so small it would be okay not to do the dissection. It's up to you to decide what treatment you want. You should exert your rights as a patient to set the course of action."

I had been curious and eager to meet Dr. Belgrad. In my estimation, he lived up to his nurse's description that he was very personable—a mild and gentle person with a kind manner. He did not hurry through the consultation. I was extremely pleased with what I observed. He conveyed that he cared, that he offered the best care possible with a minimal invasive approach. As he left the room I turned to my husband, burst into happy tears, and said, "He is the man in my dream. I definitely feel that he is the man in the dream that made me feel safe and secure." I felt elated and thankful that I had found the doctor who should help. My most recent thought about the meaning of the "two men" dream must be correct. It was referring not to a choice between surgeons, but to who would help following the surgery.

Owen was pleased for me. He knew how strongly I felt that the "two men" dream was providing guidance and how intently I had sought the correct interpretation of the dream. All along he encouraged me to gather as much information about possible treatments and physicians as I desired from any source available, including dreams. He assured me he would back me up in any decision I made.

While eating lunch in a cafeteria after this meeting with Dr. Belgrad, I felt extremely emotional. Tears came easily and I had to eat very slowly. Something very amazing was going on with this dream. Earlier I had thought and hoped Dr. Horsley would prove to be the helpful man of the dream. But he didn't seem to be the right match. Now I definitely felt Dr. Belgrad fit both personality-wise and physically.

My elation carried over into my activities after we returned home. I decided to ride the equivalent of six miles on the exercise bike. It felt good after sitting in the car and in the doctors' offices most of the day. I rode as a form of meditation, repeating the phrases: "I am perfectly healthy" and "I am cancer free" over and over. Barbara Hoberman Levine states, "Your body believes every word you say" in her book by this name. By using positive affirmations I hoped to convince my body that all the cancer was already eliminated and I was healthy.

Owen said he had awakened that morning having slept fairly well and long and feeling happier than usual. I was feeling very good about my situation. After supper I bathed and got ready for bed much earlier than usual. Owen joined me for a much needed, loving time together. Various stresses had taken their toll recently and we needed this time of closeness.

Although I believed I now knew the meaning of the "two men" dream, I felt I still needed to consider Joan Windsor's recommendations. She had urged delaying the operation in order to have Horsley as the surgeon. But I now felt certain that the "short man" in the dream was referring to Dr. Belgrad, not Dr. Horsley. I also now felt comfortable in having Swensson as the surgeon. He had patiently answered all my questions and Tony Munoz had confidence in his abilities. Although Joan gave her thoughts on the situation, she could not really know my "felt" sense of the men in the dream. She did say I was the one who had to make the decisions. The recent dream seemed to be saying the same thing when the "female friend" went her own way and left me feeling deserted and on my own. I had a strong intuitive feeling that my dreams were giving me guidance. Thus I chose Swensson for my surgeon and Belgrad for the radiologist. I did not know how much credence to give her advice regarding the dates for the surgery based on numerology and astrology. I decided simply to choose a date that fit our schedule.

Although these choices felt right, I still had questions and doubts about what basic course of treatment I should follow. I had heard the three standard forms of cancer treatment—surgery, radiation, and chemotherapy— referred to as "Slash, Burn, and Poison." This reflects the feelings of many patients that the common cancer treatments are invasive and harsh with many potentially severe side effects. It certainly seems that way to me. I didn't want to undergo any more procedures than absolutely necessary. Sylvest told me that it didn't really matter what I did on a physical level, that I probably didn't need any further treatments, but the suggestion of a lumpectomy with possible radiation was good. So I proceeded with plans for a lumpectomy while seeking more information from whatever source I could think of.

4

Facing the Knife

> Today we need to be prepared for any venture into a hospital or health care relationship as if we were entering a foreign country. Assume that you do not understand the language, the culture, or the customs.
>
> — Neil A. Fiore,
> *The Road Back to Health*

Some of the first phone calls I made were to several friends who had had cancer themselves. I listened with great interest as they described the details and their feelings about their own situations. Various people told me of friends, relatives, and acquaintances who had had breast cancer, and I was given the pros and cons about several hospitals and various surgeons in Richmond, Charlottesville, and Farmville. I was told whether the patient had needed private nurses or had a private room. I was advised to insist on an itemized list of hospital charges to ensure I didn't pay for something not used. (I guessed that person had had a problem on that score.) Everyone's experience was different. Most of the conversations were on a positive note. However, one college friend told me about a bad experience her daughter had at age eighteen when a lump had been found. She urged me to get more than one opinion and to keep her informed. One friend's brother, an oncologist, when asked for advice for another community breast cancer patient, had said that different doctors would have different opinions. I had already discovered this for myself.

CONVERSATIONS WITH OTHER BREAST CANCER PATIENTS

On Monday, February 21, I called Sandra McLanahan to tell her my plans for treatment. Earlier she had given me the name of a former breast cancer patient, urging me to contact her. Now she asked if I had contacted this woman yet. I hadn't. Sandra thought her information might be helpful should I undergo radiation therapy. After supper, I finally called her; I'll call her Liz.

I found her very open and eager to pass on what information she could about her experience. Following a mastectomy, she chose to have breast reconstruction because she felt she was putting Humpty Dumpty back together again. It was an ordeal, but she wanted it so badly she thought it was worth it. Sometime during the process she developed a second primary tumor with six cancerous lymph nodes. She underwent chemo for eight months. The doctors gave her eighteen months to three years to live. That was eight years prior to our conversation.

Liz announced that she had Sandra McLanahan to thank for her life. She had gone to Sandra for help with diet and nutrition. Her diet included no alcohol, no sweets, no juices (whole fruit is okay because it gives fiber also) and the Dean Ornish program Owen and I had been following. She said you need to feed your healthy cells so the chemotherapy won't destroy them. She stuck to this program almost to the letter.

Her oncologist had told her she stayed healthier and stronger than anyone he knew. She didn't get nauseated. She listened to relaxation tapes given to her by Sandra and music while being given chemo. She also took nausea medication—Benadryl and Reglan—which was prescribed. She said there may be something better now. She visualized the chemo as a very good, healing thing for her body. She saw it in her mind as "liquid gold" that would heal the body—"liquid gold" that would go all through the body and then flush out through her feet. She was able to cut her medication by one-half, but got sick when she cut it down to one-third the original amount.

Liz stated she thought that once you have cancer you need to take the treatments doctors present. But in addition to traditional treatments she had gone through the program of Commonweal in California twice. She, too, had had a consultation with Shelton Horsley.

She described Commonweal as a place that provides you with the opportunity and environment to help you open up and to give you a new lease on life. The program, which is led by Michael Lerner and includes group and individual counseling, massage, and music therapy, helps you learn what in your life has gotten your immune system down. Liz had gone to different types of healing programs, but she thought visualization and meditation were better than these had been. She thought power had to come from within. Mental attitude on one's part would be what would help. She proudly said she used these healing modalities every day. She mentioned in particular visualizing in the shower that she was cleansing her body of all cancer cells. She believed her new mental attitude had kept her immune system up since going to Commonweal. The program there evidently helped her understand her life dynamics and increased her self-confidence. She said her marriage had gone bad about the time cancer developed. Now at age fifty-seven with two grown children, she had been by herself for three years, divorced two years. She was very optimistic about her future.

At this time I didn't know what treatments would be recommended for me after the lumpectomy. It probably would depend on whether the cancer had spread to any lymph nodes. Dr. Sylvest thought the cancer was not likely to be in the lymph nodes, and I certainly hoped this would be the case. I did not want to have chemotherapy. In either case—whether I would have chemo or radiation—I could follow much of the same approach in regard to nutrition, visualization, and positive attitude as Liz had described. I'm sure this is what Sandra McLanahan hoped.

Another contact I made at this time was a young woman in her mid-forties who had been diagnosed with breast cancer the preceding October. I was introduced to her through the "Tumor Registrar" at Southside Community Hospital, whom I had called to ask if she knew of someone who had had a lumpectomy who might be willing to talk with me.

I met with this young woman, whom I'll call Sue, several times. She, too, was quite willing to tell me all about her experience, which she was still going through. After being diagnosed with breast cancer in October, she had further surgery done by a Farmville doctor in November. She described her procedure as being a "segmental," which takes more tissue than a lumpectomy. She said doctors told her a lumpectomy is good because it leaves breast tissue into which any lingering cancer cells can go. This is preferable to going into the lungs, which lingering cancer cells might do after a mastectomy. They removed all lymph nodes (a total of twenty-nine) on three levels. After this is done, she said, you need to try to avoid infection through your hands. You must wash your hands often.

She spent two nights in the hospital after the surgery and still had drains in when she returned home. Her follow-up treatment included radiation followed by chemotherapy. She was not able to begin the radiation for six weeks, mainly because she couldn't get her arm up into the position needed for the treatment. Since the local hospital did not have radiation equipment, she had to go to Richmond for this. She had been told her radiation treatments would last five to seven weeks; they lasted seven weeks plus two days. She had a skin burning reaction and had to delay treatment a couple of days to allow healing.

She stayed home from work for four weeks after surgery, but had returned to work by the time she began the radiation treatments. Many times she drove herself to Richmond from her home in the country, then returned to Farmville to work. She said she became extremely tired, especially three-fourths of the way through the radiation treatment. I don't see how she managed to do all she did. She had finished these treatments only two weeks before I was speaking with her.

She started chemo right after the end of the radiation treatment. Her cancer was a 1 cm. invasive cancer. It was borderline whether to have chemotherapy following the radiation. Her estrogen receptor cells were negative. At the time we were talking, she was half way through her chemotherapy treatments, which included a medication to counteract nausea. She said the chemotherapy made her feel "this is not me in this body." This feeling lasted for a couple of days after the IV was given. During this time she felt like she wanted to shake it off but couldn't. She felt tired, but not nauseous. She gave me great details on the type of medication and the course of her treatment, which she hoped would be coming to an end.

I greatly appreciated Sue's willingness to give me so much information. It helped me have some idea of what I might be facing. She also took me by the Oncology Unit at the hospital to acquaint me with it and to get the "handout" booklets. Chemotherapy could now be done in Farmville. Doctors or other technicians from MCV would come over at least twice a month to supervise. Sue was having her treatments here. If I should need chemo, I could have it done here also.

I developed a strong feeling of kinship with Sue and hoped I would be able to be of some support to her as she continued her own treatment. She recommended a book, *Affirmations, Meditation and Encouragements for Women Living with Breast Cancer,* by Linda Dackman, which she was finding helpful.

PREPARATIONS FOR THE HOSPITAL TIME

After deciding that Dr. Swensson should do the lumpectomy, I began making various arrangements in preparation for the surgery. The day following the consultation with Dr. Swensson I made reservations at a motel near the hospital in Richmond for the night before my surgery for both of us, and one or more additional nights for Owen. I also reserved a space at a local kennel for our black cocker spaniel, Cindy.

A friend who had had a mastectomy told me she had needed to have someone with her at the hospital during the night following her operation, so I decided I might need someone. Wanting to make it possible for Owen to sleep that night, I decided to ask my lifelong friend, E.J., in North Carolina if she could come to be with me that night. In an earlier conversation she had offered to come at the end of the month to help us out if I had already had the operation by then. At the time I didn't know when it would be, so I said we'd have to see what developed. When I called her with this request, she said she would be glad to come Tuesday, March 1, the date set for the operation.

Later I had an opportunity to question another woman about her hospital experience after a lumpectomy. She reported that she has not had anyone staying with her that first night; the nurses had been helpful. When she came home, her son stayed one night. Then she was on her own. The other person had had a mastectomy which was a much more serious operation and entailed a longer hospital stay than the lumpectomy. This made me think I probably could manage without someone staying with me. I decided to call E.J. to free her from coming. I'm glad I was able to do this. March 1 is her birthday. She had been willing to forgo a dinner celebration in order to come to me. What a friend!

PRE-ADMISSION TESTING

The following Monday a nurse or secretary in Admitting at the hospital called to get advance information to facilitate speedier admission on the day of the operation. She asked for my name, address, birth date, employment, husband, occupation, and whether I had a Living Will and/or Medical Power of Attorney. The reference to a Living Will and Medical Power of Attorney did not disturb me. I had no fear of dying during the surgery, and I realized it was routine for hospitals to request these for any surgical procedure. I should bring copies with me when I came for pre-admission testing on Thursday.

For Pre-Admission Testing a brief medical history was taken, blood was drawn for analyzing, and blood pressure taken. I was also given a very cursory physical exam and a chest X-ray.

Next we went to Dr. Swensson's office where I raised questions about the two procedures Swensson intended to do. Rosa said she would arrange a phone conference between Belgrad and Swensson sometime tomorrow between Swensson's operations.

A PUZZLING DREAM

As I went to sleep Thursday night, I was still wrestling with fears about the operation. I didn't know whether to go ahead as Swensson planned or to do only part of it or none of it. This question was raised in our consultation with Dr. Belgrad. In particular, I was questioning whether to have the lymph node dissection. I asked myself for a dream that would help with this decision. Upon awakening Friday morning, I remembered two dream segments. They seemed significant, but very puzzling.

From Burning Coals to a Fountain

The first part:

> *I am in a small gathering around something like a campfire with burning coals. I sense that people including small children and other creatures are seeking refuge and protection. I watch and see one or two very small children right by the burning coals. I wonder about their safety. Something (I don't know what) makes me call out urgently: "Get her out! Get her out!" I become terrified and afraid for her safety. As someone reaches for the very small child who is right by the coals, she falls over with her head going into the coals. I don't know whether I scream out "She is destroyed" or if I just think this. I don't know if her falling is caused by the person's effort to get to her or if this would have happened anyway. I do not know who it is that reaches for her. But I know no one has done anything quick enough to save her.*

I asked myself: Does this mean I should have the lymph nodes out in order to do something quick enough to save me, or does it mean that the action taken by someone to save the child (which might be symbolic of a surgeon's action—attempt to rescue) causes the destruction and therefore I shouldn't have the surgeon do anything?

The second part:

> *I walk up to a place where we are building or preparing to build and I see my father working, constructing a small pool. I don't remember much about the setting. There is no house. But it is outdoors where there is a slight dip in the ground. I see that there is just a small round pool area constructed by the time I am observing. Later, I come back and the area is much more developed with some terracing around the pool—as my father often fixed for planting flowers. There is a beautiful fountain with cascading water in the pool.*

I interpreted this part of the dream to be very positive. Various people have suggested to me that I have a strong positive association with my father, therefore this may represent my building something—my life—in the future. In one type of art therapy, one of the stages of a person's psychological development is sometimes symbolized by a fountain and is called the "Transcendence" stage, at which there is complete psychological healing. At this stage you reach a different level of awareness and the "pain" you have experienced becomes the springboard for new inner growth. Very positive energy is released and change goes through the whole person .

Thus, the dream seemed to indicate a positive future, but I was still confused. I didn't know how the dream answered my question about the planned surgery. Months later at a dreamwork conference, after all these decisions were made and all treatments were finished, I received what seemed a reasonable interpretation of this dream. At this point I still didn't know what I should do.

PHONE CONSULTATION WITH MY SURGEON

Dr. Swensson called mid-morning. He had talked with Dr. Belgrad, who evidently simply told him he had discussed alternatives, without expressing his "leaning."

I questioned the possible side effects of taking out the axillary nodes. "I have never had anyone who had a problem with a swollen arm," he replied. "I have never injured a major nerve, but I can't be absolutely sure it might not happen accidentally sometime. I will be cutting two intercostal nerves that go to the skin, so there will be numbness under the arm. This should be the only thing affected."

"I still don't know what I should do."

"Let me explain why I think we should do the axillary dissection," began Dr. Swensson.

"The standard breast cancer is 'infiltrating ductile carcinoma.' The kind you have is 'mucinous colloid carcinoma.' It, too, is 'invasive,' but 'represents a low grade neoplasm.' It is a subtype of cancer which is 'better acting' than some other kinds. The average, standard kind has a 20% chance of having node involvement. Your kind has a 5 – 10% chance of positive node involvement. It does not metastasize as quickly as the standard breast cancer, so if it does go to the nodes, it helps to get it out. In standard breast cancer if it is already in the nodes it probably has already spread elsewhere.

In your kind, if you had one positive node you'd still have a good chance. It helps to get the node out. But this is not the case in the standard kind of breast cancer. I think the risk of the axillary dissection is quite small and it would be therapeutic to get the nodes out. If the nodes are 'negative' it would be good to know.

"As to the margin around the lump, it is not a comfortable margin. Think of the breast as a bowl of jello out of which you cut a piece and know it is clean.

"Different people, different doctors might have different philosophical views. I believe I can cure it by going back in and doing these things now. You don't get a second chance. If you wait and two to five years down the road there is a recurrence, it would be much harder to deal with."

I'm not sure whether he spelled it out in so many words, but I thought he felt we probably would not be able to stop the cancer at that point.

"The other view would be: There is so little chance of a problem that you don't need to go back in now; so wait and see," he continued. "I think you have a better chance when you do the 'standard process' now than when you don't do anything and wait to see.

"You might want to talk with a medical oncologist, who might help decide other follow-up therapy. It is good to get all the information you need to make a clear, informed decision now rather than make a choice that might prove a mistake five years down the road, and then at that point say I wish someone had told me 'this' before."

This was a lot of information to take in. I still didn't know what to do. Patiently awaiting my decision, he asked, "Should I change my schedule?"

"Leave it as it is for now," I finally replied.

He ended our conversation saying, "Feel free to call me to ask further questions or to talk with someone else."

I appreciated getting all this information from him, but I still wasn't sure what I should do. I wouldn't fully appreciate until later, after reading other women's accounts of their experiences, Swensson's nonauthoritarian approach, his urging me to ask questions of him and other people. The stress of decision-making was fatiguing. By lunch time I felt very tired; after supper I was emotionally drained to the point of tears.

THE WEEKEND BEFORE SURGERY

Over the weekend I tried to continue my activities while seeking further support. On Saturday I attended a "Supervision Session" for the Mandala Therapy with an art therapist near Charlottesville. Afterwards, I went by our lot at Lake Monticello, where we hoped to build our retirement home, on the way home. I was pleased to see that there was no damage from the ice storm.

On Sunday I called the Reiki therapist to bring her up-to-date. She had talked to one of my classmates from our Level II Reiki Class recently and told him of my cancer. They both promised to include me in their prayers and healing circles. The therapist's group would be meeting the next Tuesday night and would be thinking of me and sending me Reiki.

Late afternoon I tried to get Sandra McLanahan on the phone without success. Her answering machine announced that she would be away until Tuesday, March 1. I wanted her recommendation on what homeopathic remedy might help with the anxiety that was now building. In the book *Natural Healing for Women* I found information that Argentum Nitricum is good to take for anticipatory anxiety. This was a remedy she had given me in the past. The bottle label stated for "headaches or pharyngitis," so perhaps it would help if the headache I had had for two days now was a tension headache. I suspected it was. A little later I decided to take one dose of this. It couldn't hurt.

Again the weather became our concern. It looked as if we could make it to Richmond the next day without any problem. But we worried about what might come on Tuesday and/or Wednesday; snow and ice were forecast. We decided that, if necessary, after I was released from the hospital, we would just stay at a motel until we could make it home.

THE LUMPECTOMY

We had no trouble getting to Richmond Monday afternoon, and we settled into a motel near the hospital. I awoke Tuesday morning around 6:00 a.m. and couldn't go back to sleep, even though I didn't need to be at the hospital until 9:00. I felt apprehensive as

I got ready to go to the hospital. I had been given such varying opinions about what I should do. I really dreaded the possibility of bad nausea after surgery and possible complications from the axillary dissection. Realizing how I felt, Owen assured me it would be still all right to change my mind, saying, "I understand your concern and feelings and if you feel at any time during the last hour before we are to go to the hospital that you really don't want to go through with the operation, it will be okay."

We did go on to the hospital. I checked in at the outpatient desk, and then was taken back to a little room to start getting ready. I still had misgivings and declined to sign the consent forms until after talking with Dr. Swensson. The anesthesiologist, a friendly, kind young man, came in and asked me various questions. When he and the nurse were out of the room attending to something, I burst into tears. Seeing my emotional turmoil the nurse went out and brought Owen back to me. When Dr. Swensson came in and saw how anxious I was, he, too, said it would be okay if I didn't want to go ahead with the operation. But then he repeated some of what we had discussed earlier. I finally decided I should go ahead. Three nurses came in to take me to the OR. I thanked them in advance for their help and as Swensson was leaving the room I reached out my hand to him and assured him I had confidence in him. Owen told me later he thought it was very sweet of me to do this. I told him I felt it might help Swensson to hear my expression of confidence before the surgery since he had known of my struggle to make a decision. I had also thanked the OR nurses similarly after the biopsy.

An IV had been inserted and some sedative must have been administered because I didn't remember much beyond telling Owen I loved him and being wheeled away to the OR.

I began to "come to" noticing a clock on the wall which said some time around 12:24. I was in the recovery room and was aware of other patients being with me in the large room. Nurses were milling around, attending to their patients. I saw the anesthesiologist walk by some distance away from me. A gurney was rolled in and put right next to mine. I was kept in recovery until I was staying conscious most of the time. Then a young man rolled me up to my room in the Atrium. I heard someone speak as I was brought into my room. I recognized Owen's voice, but I continued to doze off for several hours. Nurses periodically took my vital signs.

After I was brought to the room, Owen went downstairs to a small cafe in the Atrium to get a sandwich. At supper time I encouraged him to go out to dinner and get away for awhile. My supper consisted of some apple juice and a little jello.

Earlier in the afternoon I was given a shot (Demerol, I think) for pain. Shortly afterwards I began to feel slightly sick at my stomach, but I succeeded in not throwing up. This was the only hint of nausea I had. I assume the anesthesiologist managed to find something that didn't cause me trouble. I had given him the records from my knee surgery of four years earlier and urged him to give me a different anesthesia. I remembered being quite nauseated after that operation. Maybe my affirmations for several days and nights helped. I had affirmed: "I will wake up nausea-free."

Early to mid-afternoon a lovely spring flower bouquet arrived from my dearest friend, E.J., and her husband. Even before the flowers arrived, E.J. called to see how I was. I was able to chat with her a few minutes and wished her "Happy Birthday."

Owen was very attentive. I'm sure he was relieved that I got through the operation okay. He told me he hated for me to have to have the operation while I was so upset about it, but he felt it was the right thing to do. He wanted to sit with me as long as I wanted him to. I loved having his company, but I could tell he was exhausted. So around 10:00 p.m. I encouraged him to go to the motel and hoped he could get a good rest.

I woke up every hour or two during the night, and the nurses kept checking my vital signs. At one point I heard the patient next door moaning and groaning. She evidently called for a nurse, who came and attended to her.

An oncologist dropped by. We wondered who asked him to come because we had not contacted him ourselves. Maybe Dr. Swensson did; he was the medical oncologist Swensson had recommended. He announced we needed to wait until we got the pathology report on the lymph nodes to know what our next step should be.

Wednesday I awoke around 6:00 a.m. Not being able to sleep any more, I watched news on TV for an hour or so.

At 7:50 my gynecologist came by to see me and wanted me to know she was keeping up with how I was. She said to take things one step at a time.

About 8:15 Dr. Swensson came by. "The operation went real well," he announced. "Do you have any questions?" I couldn't think of any immediately. "You can go home today, after lunch, or wait until tomorrow, whichever you'd rather."

"I'll wait 'till Owen comes," I replied. "I'll discuss it with him and decide."

After Owen arrived, we began to ponder whether I should stay another night or go on home after lunch. Again the weather was the main issue. Although it was mostly rain in Richmond, we worried about what might be happening at Hampden-Sydney, southwest of Richmond. Through calls to Owen's former secretary's office, the Richmond Highway Hot Line number, and the TV weather number we learned that the electricity was off, there was ice on trees, but roads were okay. We finally decided we should go on home if I was really feeling up to it, not needing the hospital for medical reasons.

After Owen went to check out of the motel, the nurse brought the pain pill I had asked for an hour earlier and the antibiotic IV they wanted me to get before leaving.

The breakfast served to me was clear liquids: coffee, which I didn't want (I never drink coffee); chicken broth, which tasted like brine; jello, which was too sweet; and cranberry juice, which was flat tasting. When the nurse said I could have a regular lunch, I forgot to request "no red meat." Lunch came: roast beef and gravy over white rice, overcooked broccoli, mixed fruit cup, a roll, rich carrot cake, and tasteless ice tea. I ate a melba round (which I had brought with me) instead of the roll and only a bit of the meat over the rice. I enjoyed this more than I had thought I might. Owen ate the cake, plus a turkey sandwich he bought in the cafe.

After we finished eating, the nurse changed the dressing on my wounds and gave instructions for the emptying of the drainage cup. We were given a special cup with which to measure the quantity and were instructed to record the amount on a form given us. I was supposed to call the doctor if there was excessive staining on the dressing or if I had a fever of 100° or more a couple of times.

After I dressed and was ready to go, Owen brought the car to the front entrance of The Atrium. A nurse delivered me there in a wheelchair. I dozed most of the way home. Once there we discovered the electricity was still off, so we decided we should go to a motel for the night. Finding the motels in Farmville were full, Owen made a reservation at the motel in Keysville, eighteen miles to the south. We were about to leave for Keysville when the electricity came back on. We were thankful we could stay home.

Friday afternoon we received a phone call from the oncologist. The pathology report had just come in. "There was nothing in the lymph nodes and no remaining tumor in the breast," he stated. "According to statistics there might be 6–8 % chance this cancer would come back. Hormone inhibitors would prohibit only 1–2 %. They might also hurt 1–2 %. So we think it wouldn't help to take tamoxifin. It might cause more problems than the value of taking it. I think you still should have radiation. This will be very valuable. Without radiation the tumor might come back and would need to be operated on again. This is what we call 'salvaging' the person with another operation later, if the tumor returns. Drs. Belgrad and Swensson might want to talk further about the possibility of taking tamoxifin, but I don't recommend it."

After the call was completed I burst into tears of relief. This was good news. But it also showed that what Drs. Belgrad and Sylvest thought probably was true, that I would have been okay without this most recent surgery. But without the surgery I would still be wondering.

The day following my return from the hospital people began calling and coming by, expressing concern and offering assistance. After lunch a procession of friends appeared one after the other bringing food and flowers. Two had called prior to coming. One brought a beautiful fushia-colored cyclamen plant and a card. The second one brought some newly baked muffins for our supper. Ten minutes after she left another dear friend came bringing a beautiful red begonia plant. An hour after she left still another friend brought chicken soup and a salad for our supper. After supper one more friend and my brother called to see how I was doing.

A little later I called a neighbor to see if the stray cat hanging around was theirs. She had heard of my surgery and wondered if I would like company. She said she would be glad to come cheer me up, but didn't want to intrude. She acknowledged that some people prefer to be left alone. I told her I enjoy company, but I was not depressed. I also had good phone visits with my daughter, Marcia, who lived in Florida, and Ellen, my stepmother, who lived in North Carolina.

What a wonderful show of concern by so many friends and relatives. All this on just the first day following my lumpectomy. Everyone had shown the same interest and concern from the moment word spread of my illness.

Throughout the following months various people called periodically to check on my progress. I would update others when I saw them at church or somewhere else in town. One Buddhist friend assured me she would be chanting for me. Many volunteered to help transport me to Richmond for my daily radiation therapy sessions. Everyone's expressions of love, caring, and assistance were greatly appreciated and contributed to my healing.

My family injected humor into discussions from time to time. During a phone conversation with my brother in which we were discussing the possibility of my having radiation treatments, he quipped, "I know Owen won't mind a wife that glows in the dark." He also wondered, "How will Owen like being married to a tattooed lady?" At a later time when I told Marcia about problems with the drainage tube, she suggested I had "bad plumbing."

DRAINAGE PROBLEMS

At 10:00 p.m. on my first night home I became alarmed upon discovering that the drain connection at the axillary incision was leaking. I feared something might be seriously wrong. I recalled Rosa's statement earlier that the only real problem for which I might need to get in touch with Swensson over the weekend would be the tube's coming out; I feared this might have happened. Owen peered under the dressing under my arm and came to the conclusion that it was just a minor leakage. He encouraged me to relax and go on to sleep. We would check in the morning to see if we should contact Swensson.

At 4:00 a.m. and again at 7:00 a.m. the leak was still noticeable. At 8:30 I called Swensson through "paging" at Johnston-Willis. The operator who answered said Swensson would call right back. I was so relieved when he did call almost immediately. He said if a 4" x 4" pad got soaked in two, two and a half, or three hours to call him back; that at that point I would need to come to Richmond and he would go ahead and take the drain out.

At bedtime I was feeling miserable, upset about the "leaking." The bandages felt very wet to me. I hated the thought that I had to wait until Monday to get the tube out and the bandages off. Owen managed to replace the soaking wet original and replacement bandaging with a double layer of fresh pads. This made me feel more comfortable.

The next morning as well as later during the day Owen replaced wet bandages with dry ones. It appeared that the drainage was going onto the bandages rather than through the tube. Very little had accumulated in the tube since bedtime last night.

On Monday Owen drove me to my 2:45 p.m. appointment with Dr. Swensson at Chippenham. He took the tube out and put a bandage over just that area. I would need to come back on Friday to get the staples out. Unfortunately, he didn't notice the bad abraded place in the arm pit. I didn't see it myself until I was home. Although I knew the area was very sore, I didn't know the cause. The bandage the hospital nurse put on me before I left the hospital was so high up under the arm that it pressed into me, creating a red sore place. That nurse really did a bungled job. I tried to tell her there was a problem with what she was doing, mainly between my breasts, that she was pulling the tape across in a bad way. At that time I couldn't tell what was happening under my arm because the area was both sore and numb. The nurse didn't like being told she needed to do something different. I adjusted the tape between the breasts myself after I got home. If I had been aware of how bad the underarm area was I might have been able to prevent it from becoming raw.

"How many lymph nodes were taken and examined?" I asked Swensson.

"Fourteen," he replied.

"Can I see the pathology slides?"

"Yes, but I don't have them. They are kept in the pathology department at the hospital. You can go there and see them."

I wanted to find out how many slides there were in all. I asked if all the original ones were sent to Dr. Sylvest. (I believe they were.) I read in Joyce Wadler's book, *My Breast,* how her second opinion doctor hadn't seen all her slides and how a year later it was discovered that the diagnosis of the type of cancer was changed from what was originally thought. Then she had to have chemotherapy, although originally they didn't think it was needed. I planned to go see the slides when we went over there next. But I never got around to doing this.

On Friday, we had a long wait before I was seen. Dr. Swensson had been delayed in surgery. The nurse removed the staples from the incision and put pieces of special tape across where the staples had been. A band-aid was put on the mostly healed spot where the drainage tube had been. Dr. Swensson aspirated the area under my arm right above the axillary incision, which was a little swollen with fluid buildup.

"How deep was the tumor in my breast?" I asked. He gestured to show me "so many" inches. "Was some of the breast skin removed?" He made a similar gesture. "Why have I been having pulling sensations and sharp pains?"

"These are natural after the surgery," he replied. "The pulling, probably a muscle reaction; the sharp sensation, from nerves mending. These strange sensations may continue for three to six months."

When the under arm swelling became tight and uncomfortable Saturday evening, I became angry. I had not wanted to have the axillary dissection, the cause of this discomfort. Drs. Belgrad and Sylvest thought the dissection probably was not necessary, but Dr. Swensson's reasoning convinced me of the value of doing it. I cried, with angry words as well as tears. It was probably good for me to express my feelings.

After lunch on Sunday the tightness from fluids under the arm was quite uncomfortable. Owen called Swensson's surgical group at Johnston-Willis. The doctor on duty said we could come to the emergency room at Johnston-Willis or go to Farmville. We decided to go to Richmond.

The nurse in the emergency room, while checking my vital signs, asked me if I were a nurse. Since the thermometer was in my mouth, I shook my head, "No ."

"You seemed knowledgeable of the medical terms [I had referred to "axillary dissection" and "midsystolic click"], so I assumed you might be a nurse," she said.

Owen answered for me, saying, "She has read extensively."

After a long wait, a doctor withdrew 70 cc. of fluids.

During the next two days the swelling under the arm was fairly tight, but not as bad as during the weekend, not yet bad enough to need aspirating.

The following morning I phoned Dr. Belgrad's office to ask how much mobility I would need in the arm before the simulation. Earlier someone told me she had to wait extra time before beginning the radiation therapy because she couldn't keep her arms up high enough for the hour it would take for the simulation.

"The arm needs to be at a 90° angle to the body, thus at shoulder level," the social worker to whom I spoke replied. I was surprised by this response. The book I had showed the arm being held higher than shoulder level.

"Don't pay too much attention to this," she said. "Everyone is different."

I realized this, but I didn't want to go in for the simulation only to find I was not ready for it yet. I told her about the fluid buildup under my arm, then asked if this should have stopped before the simulation.

"The doctors will have to decide about this," she replied. "You should check with Swensson about the fluid build up. The swelling does need to be down because of the position of the tattoos for the simulation. These positions might change with swelling."

When I called Dr. Swensson's office late morning, I discovered I should come on in to see the doctor that afternoon. I indicated I wasn't sure I needed to come then or wait until the next day. The receptionist said the doctor would be away the next day and the rest of the week, so I should come on.

Owen had to leave a meeting early in order to get us there. While hurrying to leave, we found the van "dead." We feared this meant we wouldn't make it to the appointment, at least not on time. Then Owen discovered that the battery wire had been jarred loose; the car started after he reconnected the wire. After all this concern about rushing to get there, we had a thirty-five minutes wait before being seen by Dr. Swensson.

While the doctor drew off 75 cc. of fluid, I asked, "Is the fluid retention just accumulation after surgery or is it lymphodema?"

"Just the accumulation after surgery." I was relieved to hear this.

"Lymphodema is fluid retention in arm tissue, not at the site of the surgery," Dr. Swensson explained. "The drainage might continue for another week or two. But it should be stopping before long. If an aspiration is needed again, it can be done by your G.P. in Farmville, if he feels comfortable in doing this, or by a surgeon. You should be able to get someone who will do this for you just by asking. But if the doctor prefers, I'll be glad to talk with him about it. The radiation could begin before the drainage stops. I don't think it would make any difference since they do not plan to radiate the axilla."

When I asked what exercises I should be doing, Dr. Swensson replied with a question, "Has Reach for Recovery gotten in touch with you? Their exercises are fine and all you need. The tight feeling under the arm pit is from scarring and this will ease up as you do the exercises. The soreness down the inner arm is from the nerves."

He also told me to notify the office in advance if I needed an aspiration before the simulation on Thursday and he would come over. Thursday was not a usual office day for him.

On our way to Richmond for this appointment I noticed that Owen was extremely nervous. His whole body shook with what seemed to be a nervous spasm. Later, as we walked out of the restaurant where we ate supper, he became emotional, fighting back tears. With encouragement, he was able to open up and tell what he was thinking and feeling.

"One of the reasons I have been so upset is I feel I have let you down," he revealed.

"How?" I asked.

"I feel I should have backed you on your desire not to have the surgery," he replied. "You intuitively felt you should not have it. I hate to see you suffering from the consequences of the axillary dissection."

"I don't feel you have let me down. It is true I didn't want the surgery because I feared what would be the side effects, but I went ahead because Dr. Swensson made very persuasive arguments for it. Had we been able to know beforehand the results of the pathology test I would not have had the surgery. But we could not know this. So I was persuaded to go along with Swensson. If I had not done so and sometime later had a recurrence, we would think we hadn't done everything we should have done to begin with."

"I still feel I should have backed you when you were reluctant," Owen said.

"I might have further lamentations over the side effects of the surgery, but I don't feel you let me down. We made the best decision we knew to make at the time," I told him.

I had been frightened the morning before the operation. I cried both before we left the motel and again in the pre-op room. Something I read recently said it is very normal to get frightened before major surgery. Of course Owen witnessed this and the many subsequent times I was distressed over painful, frustrating, and/or frightening circumstances. He wished he could spare me the pain and distress. Many times he has told me he wished he could take it upon himself.

Two days later I could tell I would need another aspiration the next day. I began making calls to locate someone to do the aspiration. Finding my family physician was unavailable at the time, I decided to call a surgical group in Farmville. The doctor on call declined to do it since he had not done the surgery. He thought I should go back to the doctor in Richmond.

Next I called Dr. Tony Munoz at Piedmont Hospital near Crewe, Virginia. He suggested I try another Farmville doctor (whom he named). If he refused, I could call Tony back tomorrow at Piedmont and he would do it for me there. "I'm glad everything is going so well for you," he stated. "You did the right thing to have the operation. I think you should go ahead with the radiation. I know this is a lot of trouble and pain, but I think it is all worth it. If it were my wife or sister I would advise them the same way—to go all out."

The receptionist at the recommended doctor's office, after hearing my story, just said he was booked up to the next Thursday. I said it would take just a few minutes. I heard the doctor in the background asking what I wanted. After being told my problem, he suggested I go to the emergency room at the hospital.

When my family physcian was finally available the next morning, I was told he would do the aspirating, but he said the original doctor usually preferred to do it. I explained that Dr. Swensson had said someone else, here, could do it, and he would talk to him, if necessary. I was told to come at 2:30 and wait until they could work me in.

I was at the doctor's office for an hour and twenty minutes. When she weighed me, the nurse compared the weight to the last time I was there and thought she had weighted me wrong; there was a thirty-six pound difference. I told her that was correct, that I had lost a total of forty-two pounds. She wondered how. I gave her a brief explanation, recounting how I had purposefully lost the weight under the guidance of Dr. Sandra McLanahan.

My doctor aspirated under the armpit, drawing off 89 cc. of fluid. He asked if Dr. Swensson thought it all right for someone else to do the aspirating. I explained my situation still another time. The following Monday he drew out a much smaller amount. I was pleased the fluid buildup was beginning to slacken up.

The difficulty in getting a doctor to aspirate the fluid added greatly to the unpleasantness of the situation and my frustrations. In addition I was still questioning in my mind about the next step in my treatment. Did I really need the radiation?

5

Fearing the Fire

Don't be afraid your life will end; be afraid it will never begin.
— Grace Hansen

A few days later Owen and I continued our discussion of my medical situation. I admitted I was still upset with having had the axillary dissection. "I know it was what we felt was needed at the time and I certainly don't want you to feel any blame for encouraging me to go ahead with it, but I surely wish I hadn't had to have it." I dissolved into tears in his arms.

He comforted me saying, "Go ahead and cry. Acknowledge these feelings. Let yourself grieve over this. It isn't a bad thing to feel this way. It is a very natural feeling."

"I'm still not sure I want to go ahead with the radiation therapy. At the same time I'm not sure I want not to have it. As you know, I strongly favor alternative therapies, yet I'm not sure they would be enough," I admitted.

"I feel that Larry Dossey [author of *Healing Words*] is correct in saying there is no 100 percent guarantee that any approach by itself will be enough. Therefore, maybe it is best to use every means possible together," he replied.

My anxieties were deep at this time. I was "fearing the fire"—the radiation. Was this the fire in my dream of the burning coals? Am I the little girl who will be destroyed by the fire? What should I do?

The night before I was to have the simulation for the radiation therapy, as I was getting settled in bed, I started crying and realized it was because I was not wanting to go ahead with the simulation and therapy. Owen heard me crying, came in and asked if I was crying for any particular reason.

"Yes, I don't want to do what I am going to do," I said.

He looked at me with great concern but didn't say anything. I asked what he was thinking. "I don't know what to say," he responded.

"You don't need to say anything. You don't need to feel you are urging me to do something I don't want to do. I know this is probably the thing I need to be doing. I understand this."

He then expressed his feelings. "I feel there is a stronger indication that this is the right thing to do, stronger than the argument to have the lymph node dissection."

I appreciated his concern and understanding. I apologized for crying.

"You shouldn't apologize. I'm not surprised at your tears." he said.

Laughing I said, "After thirty-seven years I should think you certainly wouldn't be surprised."

He hoped I would be able to sleep. I did, but I had a restless night, waking up every hour or two. We had to leave at 8:00 for my appointment with Dr. Swensson and my simulation with Dr. Belgrad and his staff.

Dr. Swensson did not think I needed aspirating this time. It seemed to me that some fluid had been absorbed since yesterday. He prescribed an antibiotic to be taken for a week. He thought it was needed since I had had five aspirations and there had been some redness near one part of the axillary incision. He said to come back in two weeks.

From Swensson's office I went to the Radiology-Oncology Unit. Nurse "Pat" took vital statistics (weight, blood pressure, pulse, temperature). Dr. Belgrad chatted with us, discussing again the possible side effects. He pointed out that each woman's reactions are different, so I may or may not have them. I had to sign the consent form for treatments, acknowledging that we had discussed everything. For their records they took photographs of my breasts. Then the technician along with Dr. Belgrad did the simulation. My left arm was placed just at the 90 degree angle—straight out from my shoulder with the arm up in the air holding onto a knob during the procedure. It was not as pictured in the books I had read. Two

X-rays were taken and the placement of the area to be treated was decided. I received only two tattoos, just very small dots. I told the technician I understood that sometimes there were four or five marks. She said it depends on the area to be treated as to how many are placed.

The following Saturday morning as we were driving down the highway toward Keysville on our way to see my stepmother in Durham and two aunts and an uncle in Chapel Hill, I began expressing the thoughts that were running through my head.

"I'm still worrying about going through the radiation treatment. I'm worried about the possible side effects: possible skin burn and fluid retention. I also have read of other side effects, of rib fractures when sneezing after the completion of treatments, and lung injuries. These later ones are very unlikely. The skin burn is a more likely possibility due to my fair skin. I also like the idea of alternative approaches to healing and wish I could feel confident in relying on them and avoiding radiation. But I am not sure I would feel sure enough of this approach.

"My reading has also suggested that one should have total confidence in whatever treatment you choose for the method to be most effective. So I worry about having doubts and being unsure. Dr. Sylvest and Joan Windsor both stated at the outset that they felt I will be fine with no further treatment or with the use of alternatives. So what should I do?"

"It is very natural to have doubts," Owen replied. "We can't be 100 percent sure of anything. You shouldn't put much stock in the concern about being sure of an approach. Follow your intuition. If you decide against the radiation I will support you in this decision."

"I don't know what I should do," I admitted. "Logic says that the radiation makes sense. But some of my reading says that at times you may need to go against logic to follow intuition on what feels right for you. In a way I feel I've gone this far in going through the simulation and telling everyone I'm to have radiation that it would be awkward to not go through with it. But I guess this should not deter me if I should feel this is the correct thing to do. But is it? I don't know."

As we were driving home that evening, I put a Roger Whitaker tape in the car's tape player. The songs, such as "You Needed Me" and "True Love" are very meaningful to me. "True Love" has a line, "You and I have a guardian angel. . . ." I broke down upon hearing this, and Owen reached over and held my hand. Saturday night was the night before the full moon. The moon looked full and magnificent, surrounded by a beautiful hazy halo. At one point we watched it come out from behind a very dramatic dark cloud. Owen said it looked as if it should be in a Bronte novel.

Sunday morning I continued to think through the question of what to do. I told myself to continue my affirmations and visualizations. Maybe the best thing for me to do would be to go ahead with the radiation and believe in it as a means of eliminating any chance of any minute cancer cells lingering in my breast. Doctors and medical equipment can be God's means of healing. We do not have to do it all by ourselves. We can work with doctors and modern western medicine to do everything possible to promote healing.

I can visualize that the radiation beam is God's healing energy that searches out any cancer cells. I can think of the cells as frozen crystals which will vaporize and be destroyed as the energy beam hits them. Something I read in a book I was looking at in a bookstore suggested that one should not visualize movement of the cancer within the body, as this may suggest the spread of the cancer. So instead of visualizing the melting of the frozen crystals and then flushing them out of the body (as I had previously thought of doing), I'll envision a vaporizing, a complete destruction and immediate elimination of the cancer.

I shall use affirmations of a positive nature about my skin and tissue, such as:

- ***My skin will be free of side effects.***

- ***After a treatment my skin is burn free.***

- ***The radiation beams are healing energies eliminating any lingering cancer cells.***

- ***My breast tissue is free of fluid build-up.***

Monday I had a phone consultation with Sandra McLanahan

who prescribed various vitamins and herbs: primadophilus to counteract taking the antibiotic, pau d'arco for itchy eyes and scalp, echinacea plus goldenseal, vitamin B-1 and royal jelly. These might help me get through radiation. She said to call her if I had any side effects from radiation and she could prescribe something homeopathic to help. She would be leaving shortly for California where she would be teaching for ten days. If I needed to call during this time, I should leave a message on her answering machine. She praised me for getting along so well.

> The ability to conjure healthy images in one's mind as a means to stimulate positive physical responses in both our body and emotions is one of the more potent weapons we have in aiding our recovery.
>
> — Margie Levine,
> *Surviving Cancer*

RADIATION THERAPY

Having resolved the question in my mind as to whether to go through with the radiation therapy, I began treatments on Tuesday, March 29. I decided I should do it and look upon it as one of God's means of healing. But this did not keep me from having a bad case of nerves in anticipation.

Inner tension was building up on the way to Richmond. Not wanting to worry Owen, I hid my need to cry, then during a rest stop part way there, I shed tears when Owen wasn't with me. Later, as we left the mall to go over to Johnston-Willis Hospital, I admitted, "I'm really building up a bad case of nerves." Then I dissolved into tears as we got into the car.

"If anyone has a right to have nerves you do, so go ahead and enjoy them," Owen responded. That tickled me and I broke into laughter.

I had my nerves fairly well under control during the session. At least outwardly. But I was terribly tense mentally. I found it difficult to concentrate on the affirmations I intended to say during the actual beaming. I did manage to state silently to myself the first three affirmations I had planned to use. I hoped that now that the therapy was actually under way I would be able to settle my nerves.

The total time at the first session of radiation, including undressing and dressing, was thirty minutes. Most of the time was spent getting me into the correct position. The actual radiation took one to two minutes in each of two positions. The technicians also took an X-ray to be sure they were lining me up correctly.

The next day I asked if the axilla was getting radiation. The nurse said it may be getting a scattering, but not directly. At my third session I asked the technician about the linear accelerators. I learned they have two: one a photon one and the other electron. The rays of the photon one penetrate deeper than the other, which is used when you shouldn't go deeper. She said that at the end of my treatment the electron one will probably be used to give a boost to the incision scar area.

Friends drove me to Richmond for the second and third sessions. This initiated the very generous volunteering on their part, helping me get into Richmond. I suppose I could have driven myself. I certainly know of other women who have managed to do so. But I did not have much energy and preferred not having to drive myself into the city. The trips, made five days a week for five and a half weeks, gave me at least three hours of visits with each person each day. Sometimes we would make a detour before or after my session to go to a specialty food store or clothing store. As the time went on I had less and less energy with which to enjoy the additional explorations. Ten different women generously contributed from one to four afternoons of their time to drive me. I treasured the visits and expressions of caring and concern by everyone.

Owen drove again that first Friday. After my treatment we went to Framers' Workshop to see about matting and framing for the wisteria painting I had almost finished. I had been able to paint for an hour or more each of the last three days. Making an enjoyable outing of the rest of the day, we browsed in a bookstore and music store before eating supper at a seafood grill. My grilled swordfish tasted great.

Soon after we arrived home I had just watched a scene on TV where a bouquet of beautiful cut flowers was delivered to somebody, when Owen walked into the living room with a beautiful vase of flowers. He had found it on the back porch where the florist had left it. The flowers were from my brother and sister-in-law. Sunday would be my 60th birthday! It was also Easter. A dear friend had us over for dinner to celebrate both occasions.

The following Monday Dr. Belgrad greeted me as we first arrived, asking if we had had a pleasant drive in to Richmond. He chatted warmly, complimenting my art work, saying he hadn't realized (until he saw my slides which I had brought to show him) what an accomplished artist I am.

After my treatment, Dr. Belgrad came to talk with me about my procedure. His first words were: "Have we started frying you yet?" I said no.

"We're just getting started," he responded, Actually, I know he was really concerned because of my fair skin. Each time he saw me he was very friendly, often mentioning my art.

One day while waiting for my treatment, I chatted briefly with the attractive early middle-aged black woman who was having her last treatment that day. I learned that she had had twenty treatments on cancer by the corner of her right eye. It must have been scary to have the cancer so close to her eye. I think she was fearful that she might lose her sight in that eye. You wonder what the story is behind each person you see waiting for a treatment.

Wednesday, April 6, a week after beginning radiation treatments, I awoke around 4:00 a.m. from the following dream:

The Woman Denies Having Breast Cancer

I am with a younger woman who shows me her right breast that has a surgical scar on the outer side. I am very concerned thinking she has had a lumpectomy. I question her, wanting to understand/know what the situation is. She is very insistent that it is just a biopsy, that everything is okay. I feel fairly sure it is cancer and she is in denial. I am very concerned for her.

What does this dream say about me? In dream interpretation all characters in the dream can be symbols for parts of oneself. So, if this is the case, it looks as if part of me is in denial—doesn't want to accept the fact that I have had breast cancer. It has been pointed out—as I have reflected on these dreams with others—that the dreams repeatedly suggested I'd be okay even though I didn't consciously realize this as the experience unfolded and I was very concerned. This seems to correspond to the dream ego being concerned and denying "everything is okay."

An interesting point to note in this image is the fact that the surgical scar of the "younger woman" is on her right side. This is not the same side as mine. But if, as Jeremy Taylor states in his writings and at workshops, dreams are the "magic mirror that does not lie" like the mirror of the Wicked Queen in *Snow White and the Seven Dwarfs,* this makes more sense. When I look at myself in a mirror, my left breast appears to be the right breast of the woman facing me in the mirror.

> In the dream, as in waking reality, my inner voice refused to be silent but in this case split into a discussion between the two sides: one that knew there was a problem and one that denied a problem existed.
>
> — Wanda Easter Burch,
> *She Who Dreams*

As revealed in my journal, the implications, significance, and portent of having breast cancer dominated my conscious thoughts as well as dreams. The same day I wrote the following:

> *In a way it seems so unreal that I can possibly have cancer. There was nothing I could feel or see and I certainly didn't, and don't, feel sick. In fact, I feel, and am, in every way except one, healthier than I've ever been most of my life. Since working with Sandra McLanahan since July 1, 1993, I have followed a holistic approach to health which has incorporated various changes in lifestyle. My husband joined in this approach two weeks after I began and has been my main support. We have changed our eating habits, adopting a mostly vegetarian diet with a little fish. For the first three months we ate no chicken and I ate no bread except rice cakes and pita bread. We cooked without any oil or added sugar and read labels to exclude anything containing either. We eat carbohydrates—pastas, spaghetti, potatoes, vegetables, fruits, grains, etc., use egg substitutes.*

At first we found this shift difficult. It was hard to find recipes we could enjoy that were neither too complicated nor required exotic or hard to find ingredients. I never have enjoyed highly spiced or herbed food; so many recipes were not at all appealing. But gradually we have found good recipes. Owen is a very creative cook who intuitively has built up a repertoire of delicious dishes that we now enjoy. My tastes are also shifting. If you had told me a year ago I would be sitting down to and enjoying our current menus I would have said you were crazy. We also take carefully and individually prescribed vitamins and supplements, both herbal and homeopathic. I have been exercising much more than before—either taking walks or riding up to six to eight miles on the Schwinn Exercise Bicycle. The program also includes simple yoga stretching and a related form of stretching known as Callenetics (which I had been learning before starting this new regime). In the fall of 1993, Owen and I went to a weekend workshop to learn various forms of meditation. We have put the methods to practice, perhaps more in informal ways than in very formal ways. Since July 1, I have lost forty pounds. and have come down two or three sizes in clothing. I have been thrilled by this change and have taken pleasure in looking for the much-needed new clothing. Also I have had some slacks altered twice. Everyone has commented on how great I look. They have noticed my reduced size and a glowing radiance of health in my face. Therefore, it seems so strange to think that here I have been diagnosed as having a life-threatening disease. It just doesn't feel real. It is also very frightening to think that I could die much sooner than I've ever expected. Recently I have been thinking to myself, and telling others, that I intend to live to be ninety-five. After all, my father was ninety-six when he died two years ago and my mother's mother lived to be ninety-seven. Unfortunately, my mother died at sixty-three from heart trouble and other problems. But she had been in ill health most of her life. I don't remember when she was not sick. I must admit it crossed my mind some time recently that I am approaching the age at which my mother died. But even though I wondered if I might not live any longer than she did, I don't really believe this since my basic health has been entirely different from hers. I don't want to die any time soon. I have so much more I want to do during my lifetime. I want to complete many more paintings. I want to somehow use my art and art related knowledge of mandalas to help others. I want to use my Reiki abilities more, in hands-on healing practices. I feel that all of the reading and studying I have been doing for the past ten years, especially in the last five years, have been leading me in a new direction, with new insights, understandings, and abilities, that I am still to use somehow in the future. I don't want to die any time soon. Yet I believe in existence on another level after death. I believe it will be a new adventure. All the reading I have done on near-death experience, life after death, channeled messages, reincarnation, etc., has convinced me of this. But I am not ready for it yet. I believe there is much more I am supposed to do here in this lifetime. I have experienced great sadness and have, at times, burst into tears when thinking about my situation. Yet every prognosis from every source has been very optimistic. So I believe that I'm going to be all right. Perhaps this experience is just part of my education towards what I will eventually be able to do to help others.

Many years after writing the above journal entry I read a book, *Return to Wholeness,* by David Simon, M.D., Medical Director of the Chopra Center for Well Being in La Jolla, California. I took particular note of the following paragraph from the Introduction:

> Discovering that you or a loved one has cancer is a life-transforming event. Cancer automatically and instantaneously thrusts you and your loved ones into a time of crisis. In Chinese, the word for crisis, *Wei-ji,* is a fusion of the symbols for danger and opportunity. Although no one consciously chooses to develop a serious

> illness, many people look back and see their challenge with cancer as the most important and meaningful experience of their lives. In view of the many distressing feelings coursing through you since hearing your diagnosis, the suggestion that this illness may at some point be seen as a gift may seem unimaginable. Yet, with a new perspective, this unintended journey may yield opportunities for personal growth and wisdom that nourish your body, mind, and spirit in unprecedented ways.

The last sentence of my journal entry—"Perhaps this experience is just part of my education towards what I will eventually be able to do to help others"—reveals a first glimmer of recognition of the truth of Simon's statement. Three years prior to this I had been seriously considering what my true life purpose is, without arriving at any conclusions. I was feeling I should be doing something more or different, but I didn't know what. All I could do was wait to see what might develop. I certainly didn't know I was embarking upon the journey that is described in this book.

AN EARLIER QUEST

In April 1991, I attended a weekly four-session mandala workshop. At the initial session we were taught that mandala work is many-dimensional and teaches a way to connect to one's higher self. Anyone can draw and/or paint mandalas; no prior art training, experience, or special talent is needed. The "finished product" should not be judged as a "work of art." Its value is as a document one can come back to as evidence of the encounter.

In Sanskrit, *mandala* means "circle." Psychologist Carl Jung would routinely spend time each morning recording his dreams, writing in his journal, and drawing circles and "elaborating" them (filling them in) in whatever manner appealed to him. Afterwards he would feel refreshed and ready for the day's activities. He noticed that his drawings seemed to reflect his state of mind. He later compared some of his more elaborate paintings to what Tibetan Buddhists call mandalas, graphic symbols of the universe. In that culture and others, including Southwestern American

Indians, mandalas are used as aids to meditation. Murray Stein in *Jung's Map of the Soul* writes:

> Jung came to realize that he was reproducing a universal underlying pattern that has to do with putting things in order. . . . The mandala is a universal symbol that expresses the intuition of ordered wholeness. To name the archetypal factor that is operative in the psyche producing this goal and this pattern, Jung chose the term *self*, . . . This experience of drawing and elaborating mandalas would stay with Jung as the central experience of the self: emerging slowly, experientially, spontaneously into consciousness.

Jung's ideas of the importance and use of the mandala have been carried forth by art therapist, Joan Kellogg. But she believed that the mandala need not be limited to religious or therapeutic uses. It can be a means of self-discovery, personal growth, and spiritual enrichment. According to Susanne F. Fincher in *Creating Mandalas:*

> When we create a mandala, we make a personal symbol that reveals who we are at that moment. The circle we draw contains—even invites—conflicting parts of our nature to appear. Yet even when conflict surfaces, there is an undeniable release of tension when making a mandala. Perhaps this is because the form of the circle recalls the safe closeness of the womb. The calming effect of drawing a circle might also be caused by its capacity to serve as a symbol of the space occupied by our bodies. Drawing a circle may be something like drawing a protective line around the physical and psychological space that we each identify as ourself. The mandala invokes the influence of the Self, the underlying pattern of order and wholeness, the web of life that supports and sustains us. By making a mandala we create our own sacred space, a place of protection, a focus for the concentration of our energies. When we express our inner conflicts in the symbolic form of the mandala, we project them outside ourselves. A sense of unity may be

achieved merely from the act of drawing within the circle.

Mandalas used in the manner of Jung and Kellogg are created spontaneously with no deliberate forethought. However, sometimes they are created with deliberate forethought using specific images as symbols. At the workshop I attended in 1991, we were instructed to do just that. We were to think about what aspects of our lives we wanted to consider, what needed to evolve or be healed at this stage of our lives. Growth might be needed in any of four areas of our lives: 1. our relationship with ourselves; 2. our relationships with other persons; 3. our professional lives; 4. our spiritual lives, the meaning of our lives, the purpose of our lives.

I thought I was focusing my attention on my professional life, but I see now that for me all the areas are closely interrelated. I stated in my notes: "I have been increasingly interested in how art may be used in healing. I wish to explore what direction I and my art might take, taking into account my additional interest in helping others become more whole and to give relief from pain—physical and inner." This was the beginning of my quest.

The mandalas we drew each time dealt with our concern from different angles. After drawing the image we were to write about it, stating what the colors and shapes meant and what the total image meant. Then we were to call the image up in our mind's eye and ask it what it had come to teach us. The mandalas, in order, were to depict what our goal was, an image to symbolize this goal, what needs to be done to attain this goal, and the source of help in attaining this goal. We did not know in advance what we would be asked to do. What came to us arose spontaneously without premeditation in response to a directed line of thought. What came to me is described below and illustrated on pages 94 - 97.

1st Mandala: drawn April 9, 1991 – We were to draw within the mandala circle images depicting our goal. Shown on page 94.

The golden star is my inner Self. The hands are my hands reaching out to others. Even though the hands are my hands, by giving them various colors, I'm symbolizing I'm reaching out to people of many colors. The deep colors around the outer edge of the circle are symbols for the people in pain—in trouble—to whom I reach out.

The message from my inner self:

"The time has come to bring my talents and concerns together to help others."

"Don't just seek fame or acclaim with your talents."

At this session we were asked to write down our feelings. I listed concern for others, excitement at the thought of possibilities, frustration over past encounters with persons needing help, challenge, longing. I added: *"I have a deep desire for knowledge which will help me go in perhaps a new direction in what I do."*

2nd Mandala: drawn April 16, 1991 – Through visualization we were asked to see an image that symbolized what we were seeking at this time, then draw the image in the mandala. Shown on page 95.

White light is coming from "above"—or from the higher self within. As it strikes the crystal the multicolored rays radiate in all directions. I am to draw from the light within. Then from me vibrations of multicolors, multidimensions will radiate. Somehow my art will be used to send healing vibrations to those in need.

The message from my inner self:

"Draw from the light within."

"Radiate. Send out healing vibrations."

3rd Mandala: drawn April 23, 1991 – We were to depict what needs to be done to attain our goal. Shown on page 96.

This symbolizes that there is much I need to learn before the stated goal can be realized. There are questions in all directions: questions of how this might be done—what requirements there would be, even the question as to whether this is indeed the desired goal.

The message from my inner self:

"It is time to decide what is important in my life—time to decide if my art will go in any new directions."

"Prayerful consideration."

"Time to gather the necessary information to answer the questions."

The facilitator then asked: What must come out of this exploration that can move you in this direction bit by bit? I was encouraged to be open to listening to my inner self. We were told to put down a timeline to indicate by when we'll do this and hold to it. I responded in my writing saying: *This should be a continuous process.*

4th Mandala: Mandala for the "Image Maker" drawn April 30, 1991 – Depicts the source of help in attaining my goal. Shown on page 97.

This symbolizes the Inner Light which is within—with vibrations of all colors radiating out from the central core. This symbolizes the energy of love that is within and radiates out.

The message from my inner self:
"I am there for you."

This mandala workshop brought into focus the quest that was taking shape in my life. I was seeking knowledge regarding the direction my life should take. My inner self, which is the connection to the transcendent, the divine, gave me the message during the second session that I should "draw from the light within." Two weeks later, during the last session, I was encouraged by the message, "I am there for you." At the time I didn't fully realize just how reassuring it would be. In the same way that we did not know in advance what we would be asked to do during the workshop, I did not know what I would be asked to experience as part of my quest. I did not know that cancer cells were growing inside my breast, leading up to a life-transforming event. However, as I recorded my thoughts in my journal years later on April 6, 1994, I began to consider the cancer experience to be part of my education, my preparation for my life's purpose.

Once you find your true path in life, there is no telling
what miracles await you.
— Angela Passidomo Trafford,
The Heroic Path

CONTINUING TREATMENTS

Monday, April 11, my tenth treatment: "Libby," my technician, announced that things were running much behind. She suggested that I didn't need to wait to see Dr. Belgrad today. He could see me tomorrow or Wednesday. She assured me she was keeping watch on whether my skin burned. After dressing, I was about to leave when Dr. Belgrad came by. I told him I had been told that he was probably too busy to see me today and that I could see him later.

"I do want to see you today," he countered. After getting my charts from Libby, he took me to his office where we chatted briefly. "Your blood counts are very good," he reported. "There is no problem there. The one thing we do need to keep watch on is your skin."

On Tuesday, Libby said she needed to take X-rays again today. (X-rays were not taken every day, just at certain intervals.) The processor had "eaten" the film taken yesterday. I expressed concern about having them again. Libby explained that I get a total of 154 units of radiation each day. When they need to take X-rays, they subtract the three units of energy in them from the full treatment to give 151 units of radiation that day.

Each visit for radiation was fairly routine, except for a few occasions such as those just mentioned. One feature provided to entertain patients while we waited for our session to begin was a colorful jigsaw puzzled spread out on a table in the waiting room. It was a "work in progress." Each patient who so desired would try to fit as many pieces in place as possible. I found this enjoyable and always interesting to see how much had been done from day to day. The technician was in charge of administrating the radiation. I would see Dr. Belgrad at least once a week. Blood was drawn at the lab down the hall periodically. The nurses would check on the condition of my skin. When the skin began to look a little "sunburned," I was given a cream to apply. A bigger problem was the itching that started on the nipple towards the end of the treatments. When the itching began, I was given a Vitamin E oil to use. When the itching became frantic, I was given an aloe vera gel. It was their strongest cream to use against radiation burn. This helped calm it down for a while. Later the doctor said if the nipple itching continued with the gel, he could give me a local anesthetic that could be used on it, but it never got that bad.

As time went on, Dr. Belgrad announced I was doing very well. He said I would have just twenty-eight treatments on the whole breast and no boosters, since there was no cancer in the lumpectomy tissue and the initial cancer was so small.

About eleven days before the scheduled end of treatments, Dr. Belgrad and nurse Marie again said they were pleased with how well I was doing. They admitted that they feared I would get a severe skin burn.

Owen was able to be free from college duties to take me seven times. When he came with me, we often got an afternoon snack or stayed over for a special dinner. One day we decided to do both and had time to spare between snack time and supper. We found a quiet spot back of an office building where we parked facing trees. We both read for a while, then Owen took a nap for an hour. It was good for him to get a rest. It was a delightful time—fresh air, sunshine, birds chirping.

On Thursday, April 28, Libby asked if I had just five more times to come. When I responded affirmatively, she commented, "How the time flies!"

"How time flies when you're having fun!" I quipped back.

During the drive home I became conscious of fairly strong aching in my left breast. The aching had begun the day before and continued during the evening. I felt very tired and became emotional to the point of tears around suppertime. The next morning I called Dr. Belgrad's office and talked with nurse Pat. I told her I thought I should call about the breast aching while the doctor was there. I knew he wouldn't be there Friday afternoons. She said she'd consult him and report to me when I arrived. "Other patients have reported similar aches," she said. "It could be a combination of tissue healing after surgery and the effects of radiation. Is the ache in the breast or the ribs?"

"I think, breast," I replied. She recommended taking Advil for its anti-inflammatory properties.

Pat did consult with Dr. Belgrad, and he agreed with her recommendation. When I saw Libby, later in the day, she thought I was "well done"—referring to the reddening of my skin. She said, "If you're this red next Monday I'll have Dr. Belgrad look at it before I give you your treatment."

Over the weekend the redness of my skin did not subside

as much as I had hoped. Since I was scheduled to have my last treatment the coming Thursday, I worried, fearing I might have to postpone my treatments a few days and wouldn't be able to end them as scheduled.

On Monday I called the Radiation Oncologist Center to see if I should come on in or wait. I had a spot about one quarter inch in diameter where the skin had peeled off. Marie said I definitely should come in; they could do something to help.

When Marie looked at my skin, she thought it was not bad enough to have to postpone treatment. Dr. Belgrad agreed. But if the area were too bad Wednesday, he might decide to let the treatment stop then, and just not do the twenty-eighth time.

"How is the decision made as to how many treatments?" I asked.

"There are guidelines as to the range of dosage, but there is leeway for individual considerations," Dr. Belgrad replied. "Therefore it will be within the acceptable range to have one less treatment if it seems necessary."

Marie had told me earlier that some very large-breasted women get a bad reaction quicker than I did. When this happens and a person has a couple more weeks of treatments to go, they are likely to have her take some days off before resuming for the last two weeks.

I was given a cleansing spray and a special Vaseline gauze to use, along with the aloe gel I already had, on the problem area. I was also given a stretch net to use to hold the gauze in place. But I wasn't able to leave it on; it irritated my skin.

Each day the area of skin breakdown was slightly larger than the day before. On Wednesday, May 4, Dr. Belgrad wanted to see me before my treatment. He examined the skin breakdown, then after checking to see how much my total dosage had been by now, he announced I could stop with today's treatment. So I had my last treatment!

The basic treatments—surgery and radiation—were now completed. I was given an appointment to come back in a week to be checked by a nurse, then five weeks later to see Belgrad. The last time I had seen Dr. Swensson he said everything was healing okay. My next appointment with him would be in July; after that, every six months for the first three years, then every year. I should have mammograms before these appointments.

When I went Tuesday to have my breast skin condition checked by the nurses, I gave Dr. Belgrad a copy of an essay I had spent hours writing relating my "doctor" dream. I recounted in the essay what I have told here about the second "initial" dream, my search for the doctor who fit the description and feel of the shorter man, and my feeling that Dr. Belgrad was the man in the dream that made me feel safe and secure. I concluded the essay with this paragraph:

> *Dr. Belgrad and his entire staff provided excellent care in a very friendly, kind, and caring setting. I am very grateful. I am also thankful that I was guided into making choices that proved to be right for me. Something very amazing was going on with the dream of February 4, 1994.*

Dr. Belgrad did not read the essay while I was there. Later I received a note (written May 18, 1994) from him as follows:

> Dear Mrs. Norment:
>
> Thank you for sharing your thoughts with me. I was very touched by this little essay. It makes one wonder whether there are forces that we don't understand that are at work, guiding us in one direction or another.
>
> Anyway, this portends a favorable future for you, I am sure. I look forward to seeing you again at your next scheduled appointment.
>
> Sincerely yours,
> Richard Belgrad M.D.

While I was receiving treatments, one of the oncology nurses told me of the art show held annually at the Oncology Nurses Conference. She urged me to paint something that might be appropriate to exhibit. One evening while I was seated in the living room watching television, an idea came to me for a mandala painting. I wanted to depict by means of symbolic composition and colors the healing experienced during radiation therapy. This was created through very deliberate and careful thought, bringing together my knowledge of various aspects of human psychology, the psychology of colors, and the chakra system—an ancient metaphysical system of the energy centers of the body. I drew the basic sketch on the back of an old envelope using a ballpoint pen. It was months before I enlarged the sketch onto watercolor paper and began to paint it. I messed up my first attempt at painting this, tore it up and started over. I successfully completed the painting on December 19, 1995 and felt I succeeded in conveying the message I had in mind. It was almost two years before I submitted it for exhibition in the 1997 Fall Institute Art Exhibit at the Annual Meeting of Oncology Nursing Society in Washington, D.C. The painting and an explanation of the symbolism incorporated in it follow on pages 98 and 99.

6

Coping with Effects and Taking Precautions

I certainly was hoping for the "favorable future" that Dr. Belgrad referred to. I had undergone the knife and felt the fire and was indeed thankful not to have to consume the poison.

The doctors decided I did not need chemotherapy. The oncologist had stated that tamoxifin, often given to postmenopausal women as a follow-up after breast cancer, might cause more problems than the value of taking it. So my main concern now was dealing with any lingering effects of the treatments I did undergo and considering what precautions I could take to prevent a recurrence of cancer.

Lingering effects included fatigue, pain in the area of the surgeries, emotional imbalance, and sensitivity to noise. One of the most obvious was extreme fatigue. As one might expect, I was unusually tired during the days immediately following the radiation treatments. On Saturday morning following the completion of the treatments, I went to nearby Farmville to the art show at the Heart of Virginia Festival. I was glad I did not plan to exhibit that year. I did not have the energy needed to get ready, set up, and exhibit all day long; I hardly had the energy to go see the exhibition. The walk up hill from where I had to park three blocks from the exhibit grounds was very tiring. I really pushed myself to walk around, get an overview of the show, and visit with a few exhibitors; then Sunday I spent most of the day just resting and napping. I decided not to go to commencement at the college. By Monday my stamina was building, at least a little. I went shopping. Although I got very tired, I held up better than I had in recent days.

In mid-August (1994), just three months after the end of my radiation treatments, we made a three-day trip to Wilmington, North Carolina, to the funeral of Owen's uncle. I found myself very tired and nervous during the trip. I remember especially feeling overwhelmed by sounds. The chatter of relatives visiting in the living room became overpowering, so I took refuge in a bedroom by myself for a while.

My emotional stability was greatly diminished. Problems I should have been able to take in stride loomed large. In mid-September while trying to make arrangements for lodging at the Journey into Wholeness Conference we planned to attend, I was told we would have to stay in a guest house quite some distance from the main building where I had hoped to stay. The distance we would have to walk between sessions seemed threateningly long to me in my weakened state. After hanging up the phone, I cried—louder and longer than the problem merited. My whole day seemed to be influenced by my depression over this. Owen had both lunch and supper meetings to attend. I went out for lunch, but I didn't want to do it again for supper. I became quite emotional and unable to pull myself together. Owen kindly offered to fix me some supper before he left for his meeting. I hadn't wanted him to have to go to that trouble, but I did appreciate it so much! I was too tired mentally and physically to be able to do anything for myself or even make any rational decision about either going to buy some groceries or choosing a place to eat out. I felt better after eating supper and I was able to work on my art portfolio—photos and clippings—for awhile.

Ten days later while visiting our son Russell in Chattanooga, Tennessee, we went to see the Aquarium before lunch. Part way through the place, walking down the spiral way from the top, I felt I had no strength to continue walking. I was needing food badly and I emotionally fell apart. I was embarrassed to be crying in front of other tourists passing by. After sitting on a bench briefly I was able to continue. Lunch revived me so I could enjoy the other, non-strenuous activities of the day.

These symptoms of extreme fatigue and emotional imbalance lingered for over an additional year. I recorded notable occasions in my journal. One occurred in January of 1995 during the weekend we were helping with arrangements for my stepmother's funeral. Again I felt the noisy chaos of a family gathering. This time it was at a meal with my brother and his family. Afterwards I soaked in the tub and cried from exhaustion. I cried for my mother, for not having her any longer than I did. (Mother died when I was thirty-two years old, twenty-nine years before this occasion.) I cried for being ambivalent in my feelings towards my stepmother. (My father had been remarried for almost twenty-eight years.) Later I was comforted in Owen's arms while I told him all this.

At other times I would feel emotionally drained, but was not able to label why. But on at least two occasions in addition to one mentioned above, I realized I was having a delayed feeling of loss of my parents—my mother died in 1966 and my father in 1991. These feelings came when we were passing through Durham on the way to South Carolina to Owen's cousin's funeral and again at my aunt's funeral in Chapel Hill. Both of these towns in North Carolina have deep connections to both sides of my family, and driving through them triggered my feelings of loss. Rachel Naomi Remen, M.D. speaks to this issue and gives good advice in her book, *My Grandfather's Blessings:*

> Every great loss demands that we choose life again. We need to grieve in order to do this. The pain we have not grieved over will always stand between us and life. . . . Grieving is not about forgetting. Grieving allows us to heal, to remember with love rather than pain. It is a sorting process. One by one you let go of the things that are gone and you mourn for them. One by one you take hold of the things that have become a part of who you are and build again.

Obviously I was still grieving and needed to come to terms with my losses.

Deep emotions can be triggered years after the initial trauma. On Wednesday, December 31, 1997—two and a half years after I completed my cancer therapy—I recorded the following observations in my journal:

> *Getting ready for bed I searched my drawers for a warmer night gown that I might put on. The only other one [I can find] is one I wore after my breast cancer operations and during radiation therapy. I have strong memories related to this one. I have decided not to wear this gown again. I even began to get teary thinking about this. I do not need this*

kind of trigger, so I intend to give the gown away. Owen suggested I could just throw it away if I want to. But I think I'll give it away with some other items I'm no longer wearing. The recipient certainly will not have knowledge of my memories, unless somehow the vibrational memories would linger with this gown. Interesting question.

I can't remember now whether I tossed the gown out or gave it away—probably the latter, because I do not like to throw out things I feel someone in need might be able to use. But I wonder now what someone might have experienced because of the gown. I have read accounts that convince me that vibrational memories can linger on things. So, please forgive me, whoever wore the gown, if you felt sad and troubled when you wore it.

A major lingering physical effect is discomfort—often a deep aching and some slight numbness—which I still have under my left arm as a result of axillary excision of the lymph nodes. I wish I had not had any nodes taken out. Had I known the full interpretation of the dream of the burning coals and the fountain (discussed previously), I might have chosen not to have the lymph nodes removed. A full discussion of this dream appears later in this book.

Medical progress has been made concerning the need for this procedure in recent years. Not long ago a friend told me that it is not always necessary to have the axillary excision now. When she was diagnosed with breast cancer they performed a "sentinel lymph node biopsy." In this procedure only the first lymph nodes draining the tumor are removed and examined. It is assumed that if they are clear that the cancer has not spread to other nodes and removal of more nodes is unnecessary. If cancer is found in the first nodes, then a standard armpit biopsy (axillary dissection)—the removal of more nodes—is performed to prevent local recurrence and to learn the extent of the spreading. However, long term results are not yet available. There is some possibility that the tumor might spread to a higher node without landing on the sentinel node. In such a case, a "false-negative" diagnosis might result, leading to under-treatment. It appears to be safest for women with smaller tumors who show no evidence of lymph node spread on physical exam. According to Dr. McLanahan, "Current studies indicate

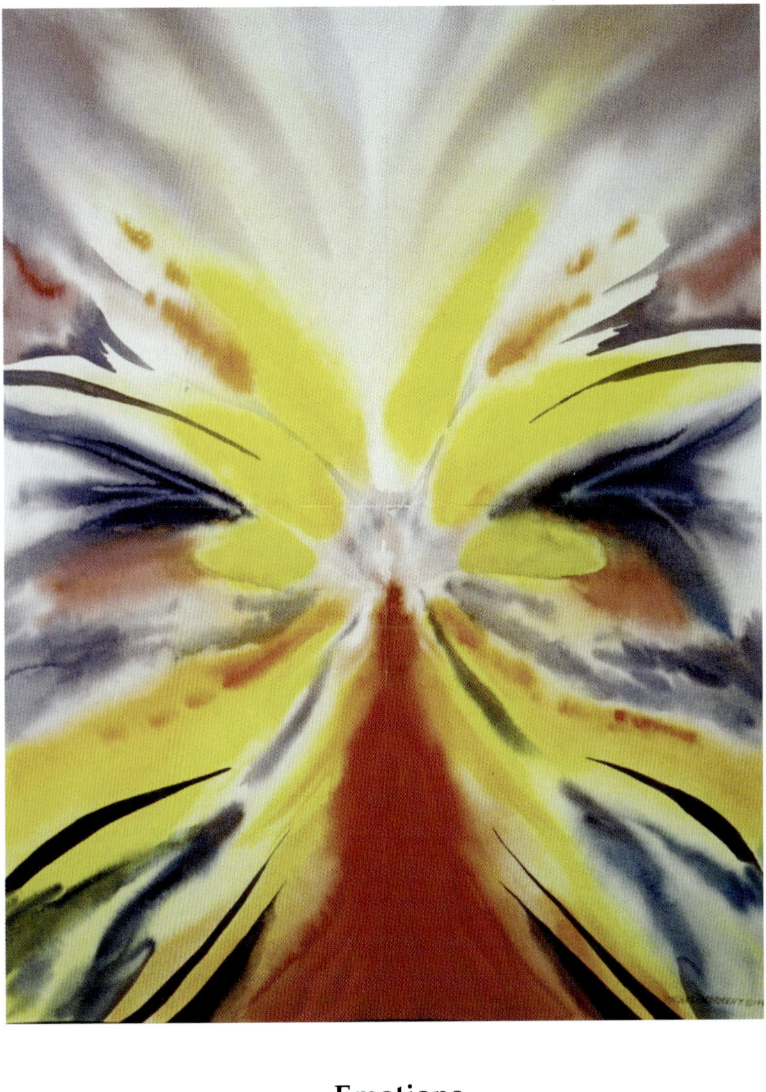

Emotions
Watercolor
21.5″ x 28.5″

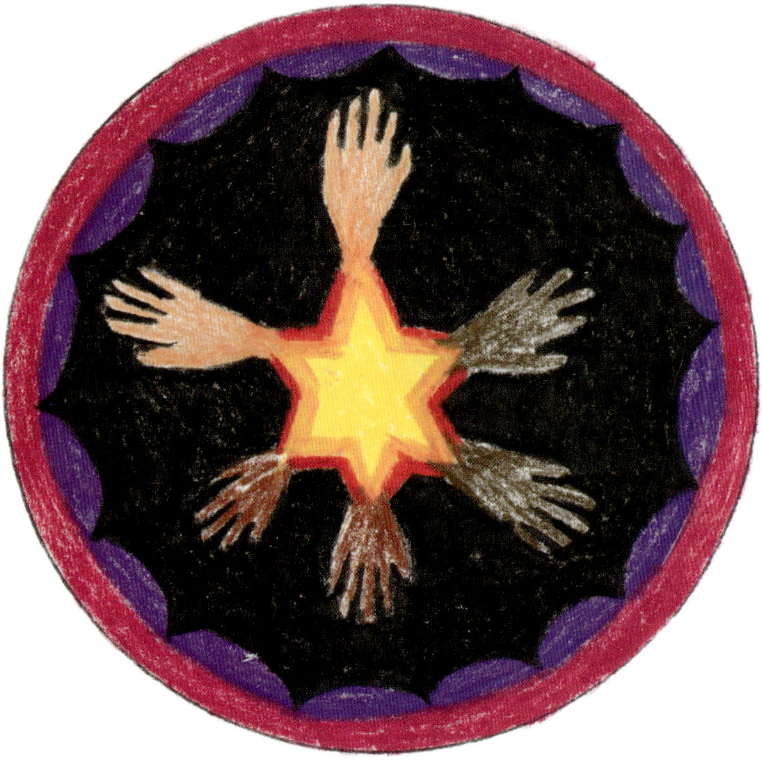

1st Mandala
Colored Pencil
5.25″ Diameter

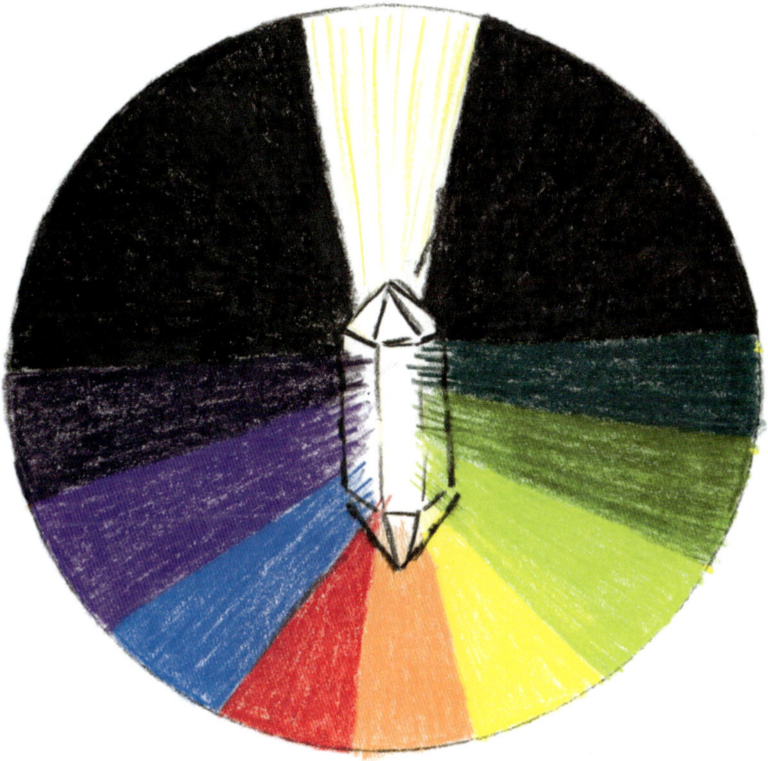

2nd Mandala
Colored Pencil
5.25″ Diameter

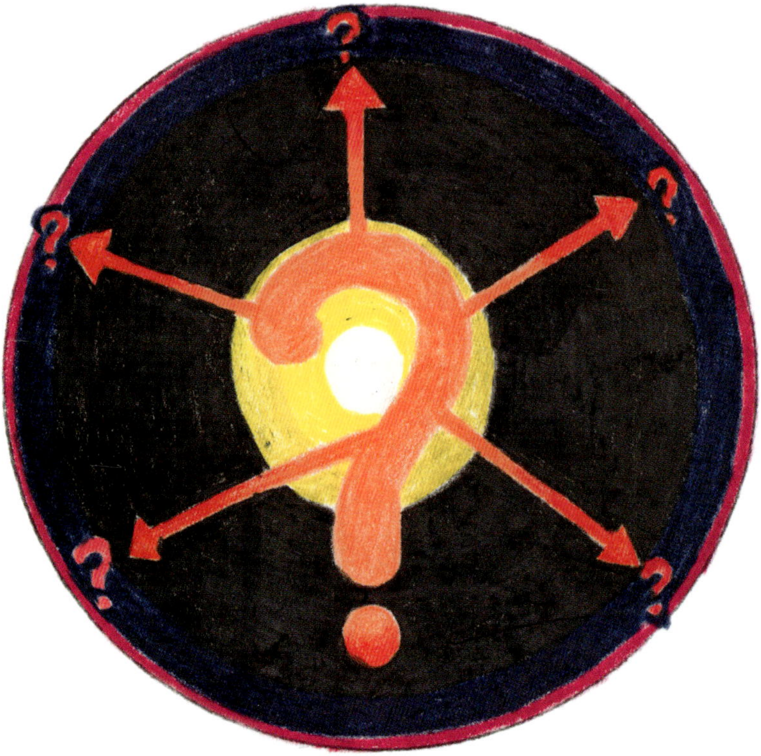

3rd Mandala
Colored Pencil
5.25″ Diameter

4th Mandala
Colored Pencil
6.25″ Diameter

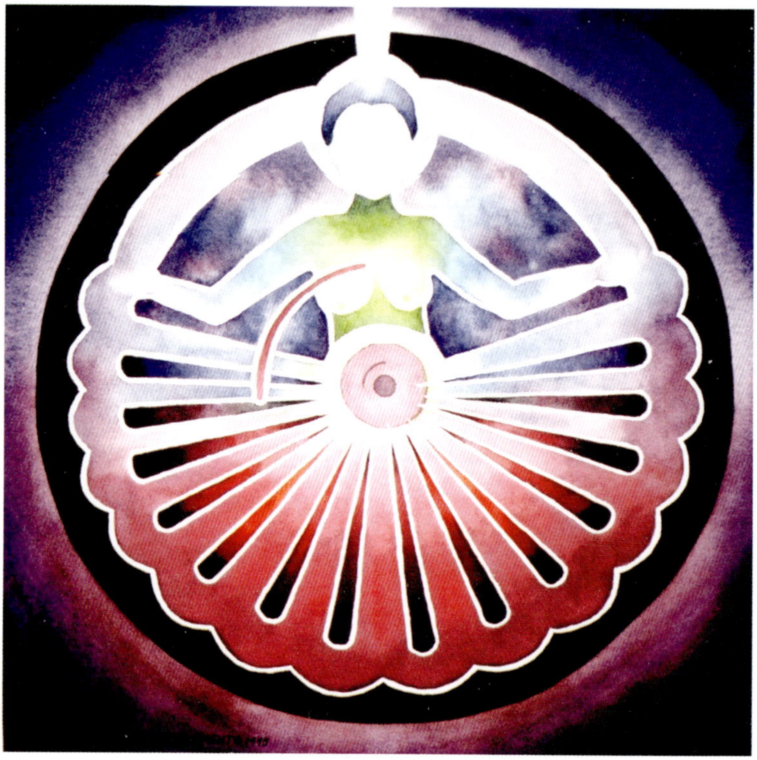

Radiation Therapy
Watercolor
14″ x 14″

Radiation Therapy

The watercolor painting, Radiation Therapy, is in the form of a mandala, a Sanskrit word meaning circle. The composition and colors are symbols for the healing experience during radiation therapy following a lumpectomy. While each treatment was taking place I visualized healing energies coming into my body through the crown chakra and by means of the actual radiation. I visualized the radiation beams vaporizing any remaining cancer cells to eliminate them from my body. The colors in the painting have symbolic meaning: the reds for radiation, anger, survival needs, and life energy; the blue for receptivity; the green for growth and healing; the indigo blue for higher knowledge; the purple for struggle and high calling; and the lavender for spiritual growth. The breast showing the lumpectomy scar is depicted three times. The black, almost enclosed, circle suggests the need to protect oneself and build safe boundaries and to develop courage needed to confront fears. But note that the circle is not completely closed. There is an opening at the top to let in the healing energies.

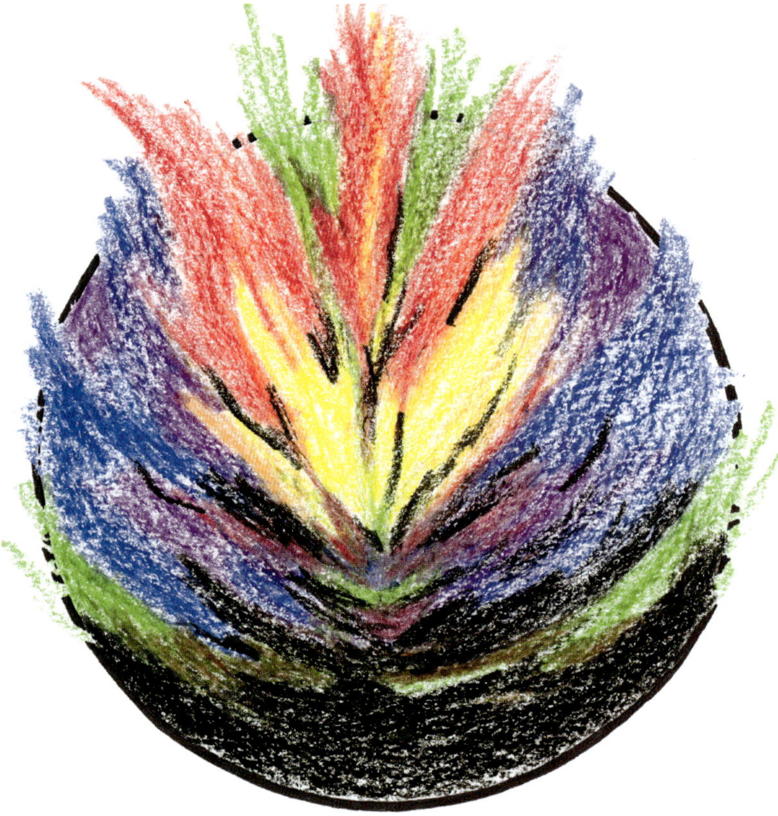

Breaking Through Boundaries
Oil Pastel
10.5″ x 11″ Oval

about ninety-five percent of sentinel nodes can be successfully located." (*Surgery and Its Alternatives.*) I wish this form of lymph node biopsy had been available for me, but I am thankful it will save many women the trauma and pain related to unnecessary axillary dissections. Some women suffer major, long-lasting pain and discomfort due to lymphedema as a result of the lymph node removal. Others, myself included, escape this problem but have numbing under the armpit due to cut nerves and experience various aches and pains for years after the excisions.

DISCOVERING HIDDEN EMOTIONS

During the year of diagnosis, surgery, radiation treatments, and follow up checkups, I had many questions, qualms, and quivering emotions. Yet I thought I was doing very well; my outlook was basically positive. But I discovered that some feelings were still buried in my unconscious. They made themselves known to me at unexpected times through my actions and dreams.

On January 12, 1995, I completely lost my cool when I accidentally knocked some cassette tapes off the bookshelves and they scattered. I had done the same thing a day or two before, but this time I overreacted; I went to pieces, screaming loudly. Then, realizing this was a way of letting tensions out, I decided to just let myself scream as loud and as long as I wanted to, remembering that Sandra McLanahan has suggested going out in a car somewhere and doing this. When my emotions were spent, I stooped down to pick up the tapes, then lay back on the rug to relax and recuperate. Cindy, our then five-year-old cocker spaniel, was in the far end of the house when I began screaming. She evidently heard my outburst. When I quieted she came in, came up to me, and put her paw on my chest and acted very concerned. I told her I was all right and that she was a sweet puppy.

> I have learned to honor the magical healing power of tears as a resource to be used for healing and inner peace. Tears now express to me all the gifts inherent in healing: humility, truth, love, peace, joy, and the honoring of our feeling selves.
>
> — Angela Passidomo Trafford,
> *The Heroic Path: A Woman's Journey from Cancer to Self-Healing*

Even though my treatments had been completed and I was told by several doctors that they felt I would be fine and I consciously believed them, unconsciously I evidently was still worried about a variety of things. Buried in the unconscious were feelings of loss—and not just the loss of my parents. On Monday, July 25, 1994, only two and a half months after the completion of my treatments, I had this dream. In it "things" literally had been buried.

I Dig Up a Shoulder and a Breast

There are some teenage males who are bullies and want to block me from getting to something. I need to get out to a field where some part of me has been buried. It seems that whatever is there is needed. I don't remember how it got there. But I'm worried that if I don't get there quick enough it'll be too late. But I have to get past these "bullies." I devise a way to slip around so they don't see me and I get out to the field. There are rows of mounded dirt, like you'd prepare a garden for planting. I go to a row at the far end of the area. Someone else is there with me. Whoever it is is probably discussing the situation with me and maybe advising me. I carefully pull back a layer of the covering. I see what appears to be a shoulder and breast. I wonder if it has been preserved, or if it will decay before it is retrieved and not be replaceable or usable. It has been sort of preserved in a frozen state and if it is carefully thawed at the right speed it'll be okay. I feel there is some hurry to retrieve it before the bullies appear. I "see" that the breast is there and can be lifted up carefully like lifting a mounded pancake. I guess it then needs to be carefully reapplied.

It seems to me I am wrestling in my unconscious with the fact of my cancer and surgery. I have lost "some part of me" that I want to retrieve. Perhaps I'm equating my doctors with teenage bullies, who are keeping me from finding what I have lost. In the dream I do find "a shoulder and breast" buried in a field. Since I had a lumpectomy, I didn't lose all my breast, just part of it. But dreams often exaggerate to make a point. The inclusion of my shoulder in the dream might have been prompted by the involvement of the areas under it. The axillary surgery caused a loss of sensation, a numbness under the shoulder on the underside of my arm and in the outer breast area. I was also experiencing pulling sensations and sharp pains. Dr. Swensson told me these sensations were natural. The feeling of pulling was probably a muscle reaction and the sharp sensation may have derived from nerves mending. The ego part of me in the dream desperately wants to retrieve the lost parts and hopes they can be placed back into my body. My unconscious needs to come to terms with my loss and my discomforts.

Both my surgeon and my radiologist assured me at each checkup that everything looked okay. Dr. Belgrad was trying to reassure me with the following note written on July 14, 1994.

> The results of your CA 15-3, the investigational blood test for the breast cancer, obtained at Johnston-Willis Hospital, came back within normal limits. I am pleased to pass this information along to you and look forward to seeing you at your next appointment.

Despite the reassurances, my dreams continued to reveal underlying anxieties. On Monday, January 30, 1995 I had this dream.

A Family Consultation with a Doctor

I'm with at least part of my family and we have gone to a doctor for consultation and diagnosis. I am in the hall and I can see the doctor talking with part of the family. There is a large glass window between me and where they are in the hall. I can tell by his manner that the doctor has discovered something serious and he intends to call all the family together to describe what he has found. I can't remember, am confused, as to whether Owen was there. He may have been there for the first consultation. But for some reason I go off to find Owen, I think. When I, or we, return, we discover the doctor has already begun his "review" of the situation. I am very anxious and eager to hear what he has to say. It evidently is something that will affect everyone in the family. I wake up before I learn what the problem is. I wish I had heard before I woke up.

This dream could be an example of my unconscious rehashing of old anxieties or experiencing the fear that things might not be as positive as I hoped. These worries always surfaced each time I had a checkup. Although I have been assured "my kind" of cancer won't return, there might remain the possibility of another kind showing up.

Before going to bed Tuesday, November 8, 1994, I acknowledged to Owen that I was nervous about learning at Dr. Swensson's on Thursday the results of the mammogram taken the previous Friday. Wednesday morning I awoke remembering this dream:

Fighting for My Life

I am being pursued by someone or ones trying to kill me. I am with other people in various crowd scenes. I have to dodge various attempts on my life. At one point I have to shoot my assailant, hitting him in the forehead and killing him in order to protect myself. I regret that I had to do this, but it was necessary in order to save my own life.

Clearly, I am concerned with saving my life. On one level this might be referring to my fight against cancer. In addition, we should explore a deeper level. The dreammaker may be showing me how I can heal myself in the Jungian sense of the word "heal," to make whole. Remembering that each character in a dream can represent a part of oneself, then my assailant is some part of myself. Very likely it is a negative animus figure—some aggressive and overanxious aspect of my inner self. To save myself, to heal myself, I need to get rid of or "kill" this negative aspect. We shall come back to this concept in the chapter on causes of illness and what to do to heal.

On Thursday I waited one and a half hours at Dr. Swensson's before being seen. The long wait was nervewracking; I became very anxious. When I finally heard the report that everything was okay, I was greatly relieved.

The next day we returned to Richmond for my appointment with my gynecologist. Again, after a long wait, I learned everything looked okay.

Almost eight months later, on June 23, 1995, I had a mammogram prior to one of these checkups. The following morning I awoke at 4:30 a.m. from a disturbing dream. I wish I had written it down immediately. But fearing I wouldn't get back to sleep if I sat up to record it, I went back to sleep without making notes. I only remembered fragments of it later. Here's what I did remember.

A Flesh-Eating Toxin

I don't remember the exact location, perhaps a hospital, lab, or some other institution. Somehow there has been a terrible contamination. Some substance may have been left out or accidentally spilled. I vaguely feel that some extra fine powdery substance may have been on some surface. Whatever it was was highly toxic. I, and perhaps others, have gotten it on ourselves. I look on my hands and see several black spots, maybe on the pads of some fingers. I wonder what it is. In the course of the "action" the spots spread and enlarge and it is realized somehow (don't remember details) that I have a fatal ailment. Whatever caused the spots is eating away my flesh and it will spread fatally. I think some others may find they have been afflicted also. We work to try to find a way to stop the spread of the problem, to clean up the immediate cause. I continue working. Others are sorry this has happened. We may know who was guilty of leaving or spilling the substance, but we don't blame this person and don't want to make the person feel bad.

The word "nuclear" or "microscopic" came to mind in relation to the whole matter. When I woke up I was very disturbed. I wondered if it was a message about cancer. Owen felt it might simply reflect my anxiety waiting to get the results of the mammogram. It obviously was needless worry; the report was favorable.

PRECAUTIONARY MEASURES

The fear of a return of cancer is recurrent in dreams and floated in the back of my mind, spurring me to consider what further measures I could take to build my immune system and guard against this possibility. I was so thankful for the help that Sandra McLanahan gave me before and during the early stages of my treatments. Owen and I both felt that the holistic approach to medicine made the most sense. We decided to learn more about homeopathy. In November 1994 we learned that Dr. Mitchell Fleisher, an M.D. specializing in alternative approaches to medicine, would be giving a lecture on homeopathy at the Sevenoaks Pathwork Center, north of Charlottesville on Friday, the 18th. We attended and were impressed by his in-depth lecture. We felt homeopathic remedies might be very helpful.

HOMEOPATHY

Homeopathy is a medical and philosophical system founded by Dr. Samuel Hahnemann, a German physician, in the early 19th century. Dr. Asa Hersoff, N.D., D.C., in his book, *Homeopathic Remedies,* points out that homeopathy "arose out of a time of rigid, and certainly primitive medical practices, where heroic therapies such as bloodletting and strong doses of mercury were the rule of the day." Offering a gentler and safer medicine, "its fame and effectiveness spread around the world." In the 20th century homeopathy was pushed aside by technological advances in medicine and the development of lifesaving techniques, but now increasing numbers of orthodox Western physicians are taking it up again, considering it to be valid and valuable in contemporary medicine and by no means inconsistent with scientific medical practices. Worldwide it is used by millions of people.

Homeopathy is considered to be holistic medicine because it stimulates the body and mind to heal itself on all levels, to regain biological and psychological balance. Since people vary widely in their biochemistry, metabolism, reactions and disease symptoms, it makes sense to fine tune treatments according to each individuals needs. To do this, the homeopathic physician, such as Dr. Fleisher, conducts an extremely in-depth, comprehensive and time-intensive consultation. He considers not only physical symptoms, but also emotional, mental, social, and constitutional factors that play a role in the patient's illness. Based on the information given by the patient, Fleisher explains, the doctor prescribes, when appropriate, "a single, select homeopathic medicine, called a 'remedy,' suited to the unique symptom patterns of the disease process in the individual. Where indicated, the doctor may also make specific recommendations about nutrition, exercise, lifestyle, etc." (Quotation from Dr. Fleisher's information sheet.)

The remedies contain infinitesimal doses of substances made from natural—plant, mineral, and animal—sources. They are virtually nontoxic, without any side effects, and work by assisting the body's natural processes. They do not cause problems, as do many mainstream treatments. They do not weaken the immune and neurological response by interfering with or suppressing body processes. Allopathic (mainstream) medicine strives to remove the symptoms of the disease, but often does nothing about the cause of the disease, which is likely to express itself in another way, perhaps in another part of the body later.

Vinton McCabe in his book, *Let Like Cure Like: The Definitive Guide to the Healing Power of Homeopathy,* states Samuel Hahnemann's philosophy this way: "[T]here is a reason underlying each of our symptoms, that something, some issue or block in the vital force, is being expressed within the being. Only by working with the symptom, by listening to the message that it brings, can the symptom be released from the body."

I went to my first, in-depth consultation with Dr. Fleisher on December 21, 1994, driving sixty-five miles to his office. During the next two years, he prescribed various homeopathic remedies and herbal and vitamin supplements to help my body rebuild its immune system and regain balance.

One of the supplements he prescribed for me in October 1995 was a bioflavenoid, pycnogenol, which is supposed to help fight all sorts of problems from arthritis to varicose veins, improving circulation and enhancing cell vitality, slowing cancer mutagenesis, improving sluggish memory, and reducing the effect of stress. Although I am no longer taking it as a separate pill, it is one of the ingredients in a multi-flavonoid supplement I am taking.

ESSIAC

Essiac's primary function appears to boost the immune system and stimulate feelings of well-being in whoever is using the tea, as well as possibly providing some general remedial value in treating cancerous conditions. Considering this, Essiac may have some beneficial effect on any cancer, both primary and mastastatic, depending on the individual person.

— Sheila Snow and Mali Klein,
Essiac: The Secrets of Rene Caisse's Herbal Pharmacy

During my initial consultation, Dr. Fleisher recommended that I take an herbal cancer remedy called Essiac, as a precaution, to rid my body of any stray cancer cells that might be remaining undetected. The remedy was developed by a Canadian nurse, Renee Caisse (1888–1978). (Essiac is Caisse spelled backwards.) According to Ralph W. Moss in *Cancer Therapy: The Independent Guide to Non-Toxic Treatment and Prevention*, "Ms. Caisse claimed the formula had been given to her in 1922 by a patient whose breast cancer had been cured by a traditional Native American healer in Ontario. Thousands of patients have since been treated with this herbal mixture, most of them at Caisse's own Bracebridge Clinic in Ontario. . . . Charles Brusch, M.D.—President Kennedy's physician—is said to have declared in 1959 that 'Essiac has merit in the treatment of cancer.'"

I needed time to decide for myself whether I felt it was right for me. I sought further information. From *The Essiac Report* by Richard Thomas, I learned that Caisse never made the formula public in her lifetime. It is reported that because she wanted it to remain freely available or available at low cost, she refused to give the formula to any pharmaceutical company, fearing they would exploit it for profit. This story corresponds with a theory Michael Lerner presents in his book, *Choices in Healing: Integrating the Best of Conventional and Complementary Approaches to Cancer,* on therapies classified as a "closed" therapies. He writes that

> [f]or some patients, the mystery of a closed therapy contributes to the numinous quality of the remedy. This may help explain why. . .some closed or partially closed therapies have traditionally attracted the greatest patient interest in the United States and abroad. . . . An almost mythological quality seems to infuse the story of why closed therapies remain closed.

Lerner then relates the mythological tale which parallels almost word for word Cassie's story as stated above. He goes on to say:

> This archetypal story of the "hero's journey" . . . often appears incredible to the mainstream worldview, but it is highly credible to many patients oriented toward alternative cancer therapies. It is interesting to note that the "hero's journey" undertaken by the practitioner of a closed therapy is often paralleled by many patients in their own journey, in which they partially or fully break with the mainstream system, undergo many hardships along the way, and arrive to find themselves in a community of believers where they are treated with the precious and mysterious substance. This is a psychologically potent process with significant placebo potential which may arguably enhance prospects for recovery, irrespective of the pharmacological action of the therapy itself.

Now several companies, each claiming to have the "original" Essiac, sell competing mixtures as an herbal tea blend in health food stores. I learned of three forms, each one containing a slightly different mixture of ingredients. The easiest form to take comes in liquid form, but is very expensive. A second form comes in packets of powdered mixtures of herbs, which you mix with water, brew, then bottle. The third form is obtained by ordering ground dry herbs which you must brew, using stainless steel pots and utensils and sterilized bottles. This seemed to us to be very complicated and the thought of such an undertaking was intimidating. Dr. Fleisher urged me to take it in this latter form. He felt the whole process of preparing the formula had healing benefits if undertaken in a mindful manner.

Hesitating to invest in all the expensive equipment needed to brew the mixture ourselves, not being sure this is what we really wanted to do, I decided to try a bottle of the liquid form called Flor-Essence first, beginning Sunday night, September 17, 1995. The following Tuesday morning, September 19, I awoke remembering a dream:

> ***The Instructor Sends Me to Get a Drink***
>
> *A man, an instructor, wants me to go down to the room where some women are serving drink. I tell them, "The man upstairs wants something to drink." I qualify that saying, "Not The Man Upstairs—implying God—but the man teaching the class—or leading the meeting upstairs." I am given something to take to him.*

When trying to understand this dream, I wondered if the instructor of the class who sends me to get him something to drink is Dr. Fleisher. Is this referring to his urging me to take Essiac? In the dream it's not stated that it is for me. I'm to go get *him* some drink. But I think maybe it is meant for me. It does seem that my unconscious is working on the question of whether to follow instructions. It does not tell me that I should take the drink myself. Dreams don't tell us what to do; they will give us suggestions, then it's up to us to make our own decisions among possible choices. This dream does show that the "instructor," maybe an instructing M.D., is sending me to get the drink.

The Flor-Essence tasted awful. I knew I wouldn't want to take it for the prescribed two years Dr. Fleisher recommended. In one way we were glad since it was so expensive. We decided to get enough equipment to make the brew. We bought two stainless steel pots and the various utensils we would need and had a druggist order a carton of the necessary brown bottles. Next we bought the packets of the powdered mixture, thinking this would be easier to do than the bulk herbs. Fighting our own resistance and fear of the undertaking, we brewed one batch. I didn't like the taste or the smell of the herbs in this prepackaged form, so we finally ordered the bulk herbs.

Friday evening, October 29, 1995, we began brewing the Essiac from the bulk mixture. The cooked mixture had to sit overnight before straining and bottling it. Saturday morning we discovered we needed a still larger pot for the sterilizing of the bottles and equipment. What we had used the one time before had worked because we made a smaller quantity. This time we needed more bottles. Not able to find a large enough pot locally, we made the fifty-mile trip to Lynchburg to find one at a store at the mall.

It was a beautiful fall day. Leaves on the trees were finally getting colorful. On the way over and back we listened to Marion Woodman's tape, *Dreams: Language of the Soul,* on the meaning of dreams. Woodman's words are very insightful; the tape is one of the best on the subject we have heard yet. Owen said the joy of the drive while listening to the tapes was worth the trip over.

We began the bottling process as soon as we got home. We ended up with fourteen bottles of the brew this time, which would last six or seven weeks. Standing for an extended period really tired me out. And this was a year and a half after treatments!

In the weeks immediately following the beginning of our brewing Essiac, I still had doubts about preparing and taking the Essiac for the next two years. Saturday evening, November 17, 1995, I read the first thirty pages in Virginia M. Soffa's *The Journey Beyond Breast Cancer.* Then before going to sleep I posed the following dream incubation question: What further measures can I take, what more can I do to further insure that I have gotten rid of the cancer and will not have a recurrence?

I awoke Sunday morning remembering the following dream:

The Game of Forced Combat

I am with a group of people—not sure whether male and female, or just female. I think the latter. We are told that we must participate in a kind of combat game that will take place in what seems to be an auditorium. I do not want to participate and try to figure out how I can avoid doing it. Other women go in—maybe they are called in—and for awhile I have hope that I won't be called. But I do get made to go on in. The combat seems to be a "shoot-out," western fashion. I stand to one side observing and trying to keep out of the way. Before I was called in, I may have gone down a hall away from the auditorium to a bathroom as a way of "making myself scarce"—not

> *there to be called. After being in the combat area awhile, I discover that we are allowed "time out" to go out to the bathroom. The bathroom is a strange mixture of standard and primitive fixtures. There are some regular commodes and some baskets which we use. I think I keep trying to find one which is clean enough to sit on. Each one I try is very messed up with "water" splatters, etc. I finally select one of the more primitive ones and sit. We, the women there, decide to sit as long as possible to prolong our reprieve from the forced combat. After awhile the <u>men</u> supervising this combat come looking for the women. They have become suspicious of our delay and come to find us. They—or at least one—stand watch to see if we are actually using the facilities. For awhile we prove we are still using the facilities. But finally we are forced to go back to the place of the shoot-out. This time I must participate. I decide I'll do what is needed to win the game, but without actually hurting the other players. It becomes something akin to such a game—a mock combat—I saw a bit of on T.V. yesterday in which the players shot the opponents with a liquid color which signified a hit, but, of course, was not actually hurtful. In the dream I may have tapped the opponent in some way and this signified a hit and the player withdrew from the game. Fairly rapidly I "tapped off" my opponents and won the game.*

I had forgotten my incubation question until mid-afternoon Sunday after reading approximately forty more pages in Soffa's book. I read to page seventy-two and put the book aside after reading the following:

> While writing the chapter "Strengthening the Immune System," I had a dream. I think dreams can sometimes reveal what we are trying to comprehend. Understanding my role in my healing was one question I could not resolve.

At this moment the memory of my incubation question returned. A possible meaning also came at this time. I had not given it much thought beforehand. In these pages of Soffa's book, she points out how doctors (probably mostly male) have controlled or seemed to want to control the course of treatment for breast cancer. She says the only way she could get the doctors' approval on the course of treatment was to do exactly what they wanted. But she felt that she needed to follow her own intuition and the researched knowledge, which told her that the common prescribed methods of treatment had serious potential side effects and questionable long-term benefits. However, she knew she could only base her decision on the best information available and she expected the doctors to do the same. She states:

> This information provided me with the lifeline I needed to feel I was doing everything possible to stay alive. The facts forced me to be objective and confront my fears. Once I accepted that the worst that could happen was that I would die, no matter who made the final treatment decision, I also realized that the doctors didn't have any special tricks or wisdom to significantly change the course of this disease. My future really did depend on me.

I find that much of what Soffa says resonates within me and finds acceptance in my thoughts and feelings. Here's a paragraph:

> Questions seemed to be posed by my invisible inner teacher on one day, then I investigated the answers until I had an understanding of that aspect of the problem. I followed these clues and later integrated the answers into an elaborate healing plan for myself, a plan that was based as much on scientific data as on spiritual guidance. I required confirmation for what I was being led to see and to know. I was unwilling to just accept the spiritual teachings without substantial medically documented background. No matter how much more information I demanded to know, I continued to be led to the right periodicals, books, and experts. Each contained one part, and none had the complete solution.

This has been my experience. Time and time again I am led to just the right book on the shelves in a bookstore when I need the information it contains.

So, here's what I think the forced combat dream may be saying on one level:

The men (doctors) make the women (probably breast cancer patients) go into the auditorium (hospital or clinic) for a western style shoot-out (western medicine) whether they want to or not. I stand aside observing the other women being called in, hoping I won't be called in, but I am. The other women and I try to find a way to avoid the combat, but we are made to participate. We are given "time-out" to go to the bathroom (to get rid of toxins and other wastes). The bathroom is a strange mixture of *standard* and *primitive* fixtures (standard and primitive methods of getting rid of toxins). Each one is messed up (not good or really satisfactory on the surface), but I finally pick a more primitive one (perhaps a homeopathic method or Essiac). Back in the "mock combat" (fighting cancer), I do things that cause my opponents (the cancer cells within me) to withdraw from the game (from me) without actually being hurtful to the other players (the other parts of me that shouldn't be harmed). I win the game.

On another level, perhaps it is speaking archetypally—of men trying to control women in a patriarchal society. During the weekend of March 21–22, 1997, Jeremy Taylor led a dream workshop at the Unitarian Church in Richmond, Virginia. Owen and I both attended the lecture Friday evening, then I attended the all-day workshop on Saturday. This dream of mine of the game of forced combat was one of the dreams discussed. One of Jeremy's concluding thoughts concerning this dream was that it might be suggesting that I am being called to do something to help women. At the time this notion seemed beyond my scope and understanding.

It was on September 19, 1995, exactly two months before I had the dream of the game of forced combat when I had the dream of the instructor sending me to the basement to get something to drink. At the time I thought it probably was showing that my doctor was urging me to take the herbal brew, Essiac, and my subconscious was working on the question of whether to follow his instructions. I agree in essence with Virginia M. Soffa who pointed out in her book how doctors (probably mostly male) have controlled or seemed to want to control the course of treatment for breast cancer. But I was very fortunate with the doctors I consulted during most of my treatment. They gave me their opinions, many of them being contradictory of each other, and then allowed me to choose my own path. Sometimes it was hard to make those decisions, often because of the conflicting advice and the knowledge I gained through reading about the possible side effects of various treatments.

This dream of September 19 was the fourth dream in a series of four dreams. Since all dreams of the same night are probably dealing with the same theme, but from different perspectives, I think the other three might have been giving additional suggestions for improving my health, in the aftermath of cancer. Let's look at each one in turn. The first dream stated:

The Instructor Doesn't Respect My Desire for Privacy

I am evidently away from home, attending a meeting or visiting somewhere. At some point I'm in my room which adjoins a public room, maybe where the meeting is being held. I don't remember the details. I'm undressed. Someone wants to come in, but I tell him to stay out, I'm undressed. A second time this happens, the person who I think is the instructor or leader of the meeting just walks on in, not respecting my desire for privacy. I'm standing there naked. It does not faze him. I may decide it doesn't matter.

This first dream in the series has "the instructor" barging into my room even though he has been told that I desire privacy. If the instructor represents the doctor, it seems my subconscious is showing me that I feel the doctor in his enthusiam is invading my private space. In the dream, I am standing naked before him, but this doesn't faze him. It is true that in the initial interview with a homeopathic doctor you "bare yourself" psychologically, revealing everything about yourself in order for him to know how to treat your situation. In the dream my nakedness didn't faze him and I "may decide" it doesn't matter. Self-revelation, whether physical or mental, is a natural part of a doctor's practice. So in one sense it shouldn't matter to the patient. It is also true that this particular doctor believed so strongly in his approach and ideas that he might seem insistent in urging acceptance of a form of treatment. Dreams often exaggerate to make a point. Perhaps by having the "instructor" walk in on me in this manner (when I'm not dressed or ready to receive anyone), my dreammaker is pointing out that I am not yet ready to accept the doctor's recommendations.

The second dream:

I Don't Want to Sleep in a Bed Full of Fleas

As I'm getting out of bed one morning, I notice that the bed is infested with tiny bugs. I think I take them to be fleas. I'm horrified. I even find a couple of them crawling on my chest between my breasts. Most of them are down near the foot of the bed. I get out quickly and go to my closet to get clothes to get dressed. I think later it's discovered that there are many up under the bed.

A friend offers to take me with him when he leaves to go to Nashville (which is east of where the action of the dream is taking place). He is to leave right away. I decline, saying we (Owen and I) will leave the next day.

But a little later I decide I can't stay through another night. I don't want to sleep in that bed with all the fleas again. It's after I have declared this that another woman comes in, maybe preparing to take over the room, and this is when it is discovered that the fleas are under the bedding. I tell Owen I want to leave before another night in the bed with the bugs. I might as well have gone on with our friend. But I didn't want to do that. I thought I wanted to wait 'till the next morning. But the desire to leave becomes most urgent.

This dream is dealing with my breast cancer from a different angle. I discover bugs in my bed and even between my breasts. (This suggests that this has something to do with the breast cancer.) On further reflection, I believe that, instead of fleas, the bugs were simply bed bugs. This is a very graphic way of showing that something is "bugging" me. Wilda B. Tanner has suggested in *The Mystical Magical Marvelous World of Dreams* that bed bugs "would most likely represent irritations that creep up on you when you are asleep, unaware, unknowing, not realizing the damage until it is already done." I decide I must leave as soon as possible; I don't wish to spend another night in that bed with the bugs. In order to remain healthy I need to get away from things that are bugging me. This does fit my situation. I had developed an urgent feeling that for personal reasons I needed to have a change in my environment. I needed to get away from things that "bugged" me. Whether I realized it or not at the time, I needed to be in a new place, away from old assumptions and expectations of what was important in my life, to a place where I could begin life anew, where new avenues might open.

The third dream tells me something else about my cancer. Here's the dream:

I Have On the Wrong Color Robe

At some point I'm to attend some meeting, or maybe a church service. I have on a black choir robe. I go to a doorway to go in and something is wrong. I'm not sure whether I have come to the wrong door. I think I learn that I have on the robe for the Sunday morning service—or at least a different service (from the one just about to take place)—that the robe for this service is a purple one. I see some people with purple robes on inside the sanctuary.

I believe the significant elements in this dream are the colors of the robes. The color black usually denotes the unknown, the mysterious, darkness, even death, especially when associated with fear or uncertainty. Purple can be a symbol of royalty, of oneness with God, devotion, healing abilities, great spiritual powers. As the dream begins I'm wearing a black robe. I am experiencing the unknown, the mysterious, and even the fear of death. I feel that the dream is saying I should not have on the black robe of death; I'm not supposed to die at this time. The purple robe of healing abilities and great spiritual powers is what I should wear.

As has already been stated above, in the fourth dream my subconscious is working on the question of whether to follow the doctor's instructions.

This series of dreams gives me various ideas to contemplate. They tell me not to think I'm going to die now. I should put on the robe of healing abilities and spiritual strength and vitalities, then go join others in the sanctuary for service. There are various ways to gain and maintain health and wholeness. I need to consider them carefully and make my choices without feeling pressured by others, then follow up with appropriate action.

By the fourth time we made the brew, near the end of January 1996, we had gotten past our fear of the process and were pleased with the ease with which we did the "Essiac operation." We continued this undertaking through the summer of 1997. I was still taking it when I had the following dream on Monday, May 19, 1997.

I Want to Sweep Away the Dead Bugs

I am in a house we recently moved into. It is not our "real-life" house. I am sweeping a very large closet. I note that there are no "objects" stored or hanging in the closet. But there are a moderate number of bugs scattered around on the floor. I have the feeling, in remembering, that they are dead bugs. I want to sweep out the closet to get rid of the bugs in case I need to use the closet.

I completed my formal treatments for the breast cancer three years before having this dream and had been taking the Essiac for almost two years. Now my subconscious is saying I am making sure I have done everything possible to clear away even dead bugs to make available new space in my home, my life. If the bugs represent cancer cells, it looks as if they are no longer living. I am, in waking life at the time of this dream, taking the Essiac hoping to flush out any lingering cancer cells. If the bugs are the bed bugs, the stressful irritations in my life, that I urgently desired to leave behind two years ago, they, too, are dead. We moved to our new home near Charlottesville ten months before I dreamed this dream. But I'm still sweeping the remnants of the bugs out of my life.

The last batch of Essiac we made was with herbs from a new shipment. We were surprised to see how coarse some of the ingredients were this time, but went ahead and used them. Not many days later the bottled mixtures began to thicken and seemed to be going bad. The odor coming from the pot while it was brewing had been unpleasant. This was different. Before, I always enjoyed the aroma wafting from the pot. It had seemed very healthful. Not this time! I took a bottle of the brew with me to my appointment with Mitchell Fleisher on August 29, 1997. I wanted him to tell me if it was still usable. He pronounced it okay, but suggested we could strain it through a filter paper to get rid of the slime if we so desired. He also suggested grinding the burdock root in a dry blender.

However, I decided to throw out the remainder of this last batch. Feeling I had probably gotten the basic benefit of this remedy and thinking this new dry mixture had obvious problems we would have to deal with, I decided not to make any more.

MEETING MICHAEL LERNER

Eight months later, now living near Charlottesville, I learned that Michael Lerner, Ph.D., author of *Choices in Healing,* president and founder of Commonweal, a health and environmental research institute in Bolinas, California, and co-founder of the Commonweal Cancer Help Program, would be talking to doctors, nursers, staff, and the general public on April 21 at the UVA Cancer Center. I was invited by the Director of Community Relations for the UVA Cancer Center to come to the lecture and also to join a smaller group of cancer patients talking with Michael Lerner prior to the lecture. I was pleased and excited by this opportunity. The Commonweal Cancer Help Program was where Sandra McLanahan's patient whom I mentioned earlier had gone. I was eager to meet Michael Lerner.

On April 21, 1998, I went to the UVA Cancer Center to hear Dr. Lerner at the Cancer Support Group mid-morning and the general lecture ("Grand Rounds") at noon. At the Cancer Support Group I was surprised to see an acquaintance who had bought a painting of mine many years ago when I still lived at Hampden-Sydney. I learned that she had had breast cancer twice, but was okay at the time of this writing. She announced during self introductions that she thought she recognized me, that she had bought a beautiful painting from me fifteen years ago entitled *Shall We Gather by the River?* When Michael Lerner began his talk to the support group, he said he was impressed by the title and thought it appropriate for our gathering that morning, that we were gathering by the river of life. During the question and answer period I had the opportunity to ask him his opinion of Essiac. He said he knew it would do no harm and might help and he is in favor of using any complementary therapy that a patient feels will be helpful.

Just before Michael Lerner began his speech at Grand Rounds, the Swami Satchidananda, followed by an entourage from Yogaville, walked into the auditorium. Dr. Lerner told the audience that the Swami had helped him fifteen or more years ago when he needed help. He attributes his program and Dean Ornish's to what they both learned from the Swami. Michael mentioned he is a friend of Sandra McLanahan and Rachel Naomi Remen. Afterwards I went up to him and said I was interested to hear this, that I gave Sandra McLanahan credit for stopping my cancer in its tracks and then told him how. Michael said she was there. I was surprised; I had not spotted her. He pointed her out and I went over and greeted her. She said it had been a long time and she was glad to see me. She introduced me to the Swami, saying I was one of her patients. I shook his hand and said I was glad to meet him. When I told Sandra I was thinking about writing a book, she encouraged me to do so and said it could be very helpful to others. It would be three years, during which I would take several writing workshops and read extensively on writing memoirs, before I felt ready to begin writing.

> I believe that people who are inclined to fight for life with cancer using whatever combination of conventional and complementary therapies that makes sense to them are wise to do so.
>
> — Michael Lerner,
> *Choices in Healing*

7

Discovering Contributing Factors

We cannot change the past that presented us with the challenge we are facing, but we can reinterpret the experience from the perspective of life as a learning journey.
— David Simon, M.D.,
Return to Wholeness: Embracing Body, Mind, and Spirit in the Face of Cancer

No one knows with any certainty what factors contribute to breast cancer. I encountered many theories during my journey, and I will explore these through a series of dreams I had during the year following the radiation therapy. These dreams give clues as to what was going on inside of me.

In the dreams, I encountered snakes. In ancient Greek and Roman cultures the snake was a symbol for healing. This connection has been carried over into present times by the current medical profession with its symbol, the caduceus—two intertwined snakes on Hermes' staff. The first dream of this series was on Friday, July 15, 1994.

Picking Up a Copperhead

I'm outside in a wooded area. I think I am concerned about there being snakes around. I may hear something or see something and pick it up. Sure enough, I see that it is snake. I know it could possibly bite me (I think this) while I'm holding it up to look at it. I may be trying to hold it

> *in such a way it won't do so. But it does bite me on my right hand near the knuckles. This is the hand I'm holding it by. I next wonder what to do with it to get rid of it. If I let it go, it'll be loose in the woods and could bite someone else; but I don't think of killing it, just getting it out of my hand so it won't bite it again. So I simply drop the snake. I assume it slithers away. I try to suck my hand to get the venom out and I go to find a telephone to call for help. The snake is rather small and not very long, not more than two feet, and I realize or think, in thinking about the dream, that it is a copperhead. I hear the word in my mind.*

Ted Andrews in his book *Animal-Wise* states, "All venomous animals teach us something about the toxicity and poisons in our life. They help point to paths of healing for us. . . . They sometimes appear to awaken our own innate healing energies and abilities." I should consider what I might learn from the snake. I was already aware that I feared my treatment might be a snake-in-the-grass that could harm me. Since dreams come to tell us things we don't already know consciously, what is this trying to tell me? Referring to known characteristics of snakes, Andrews explains:

> When encountered, many poisonous snakes will alert and warn, and even move out of the way if they feel they will be disturbed. The copperhead rarely moves on. It will stand its ground, expecting the intruders to go around it. If disturbed, it will attack rather than move. The copperhead brings a message of standing one's ground, even if only based upon a "feeling." And if need be, do not hesitate to strike in defense of oneself. In time, that feeling will prove itself out and standing your ground will be confirmed as having been the right thing to do. . . . When the copperhead appears, it is usually an indication we need to get more assertive and aggressive in our healing and other activities.

As the messenger, the copperhead is telling me to stand my ground, to stand by my feelings about various healing procedures. They probably will later be confirmed as being right. Since the radiation treatments had been completed by this time, I decided to apply this information and follow my intuitive, gut feelings about future treatments and preventative measures.

Even at this stage of my experience I still needed to ask, "What needs to be healed?" My first response was the cancer, but I also questioned what in my life may have contributed to my illness. What were the poisons and toxins in my life that led to what happened? I don't want to be bitten by the poisonous snake a second time. I want to let go of this possibility. What changes might promote healing and prevent further problems? The snake renews itself by shedding its old skin. New growth is possible only after shedding—shedding one's old beliefs and ways—to embrace a new path in life, possibly one of discovering one's own innate healing energies and abilities.

Ten months later, Tuesday, May 30, 1995, I had another dream in which I am bitten by a snake.

Another Snake Bite

> *To complete my "journey" from wherever (I don't remember where), I plunge into a river and swim to the far bank. As I pull myself up onto the far side I'm bitten on my little finger of my left hand. I look and see two sets of fang marks. I call for help, knowing I need immediate medical attention. A woman, maybe in a house a short way from the water, hears me and calls to me. I think I have seen a man go by who I believe is a doctor. I tell the woman to get him immediately. I wake up before more happens.*

Plunging into a river can be a metaphor for going into one's personal unconscious. I am doing this as I continue my "journey," the journey of life. Studying my dreams is one means of doing this. They can show me the toxins in my life and what changes I need to make that can be healing. This is a quest and I am being reminded to keep at it. I did not realize it at the time, but the quest is also the one begun back in 1991 at the Mandala workshop: What more am I supposed to be doing to fulfill my mission in life? Evidently I don't have all the information I need yet because I encountered a snake again. But I am to be helped by a woman and a man, who represent parts of my inner self. The woman—my inner feminine, nurturing and creative attributes—lives near water, often a symbol for feelings and emotions. I am calling to her to find the man, my inner masculine, thinking, assertive, and aggressive attributes, and in this dream a doctor, my inner healer. In the previous snake dream, the snake called on me to stand by my feelings and to be more assertive and aggressive in my healing and other activities. Together the inner feminine and inner masculine will help me.

It is also interesting to recall the first of the "initial dreams" after I received my diagnosis. In it I feared a woman was drowning after either jumping or falling into water. When she went under the water and didn't immediately come back up, I thought someone needed to jump in to rescue her. My interpretation at the time was that I (my ego) was observing myself (the woman) in danger from the cancer which had just been diagnosed. I was relieved when the woman resurfaced and did not drown. I was encouraged by this and hoped this meant I was not going to die from the cancer. What I did not fully comprehend or think through at the time was the dream's fuller meaning. After going into the water—into one's unconscious and learning from what might be observed there—the woman comes up on her own accord and doesn't seem to need more help. This is saying that I will be okay without outside help; I can find healing powers within myself. This is what Vernon Sylvest kept telling me.

Six months after the second snake dream, on Monday, December 28, 1995, I had this dream:

> ***Being Aware of a Snake Near Our Path***
>
> *I am outside walking with someone, a friend. We see our destination up ahead of us and there is a passageway to our left through which we need to walk on our way. There is a thick covering of leaves on the ground. As I look down I see, partially exposed and partially under the leaves, what looks like a snake with a diamond pattern. I warn the person with me that we must be very careful where we step. But I evidently did not say we must not go on past where I have seen the snake.*

In this dream I am aware of the presence of a rattlesnake, but am not harmed by it. The dream shows I am intent upon continuing on my path and I can see my destination ahead. I am aware of the snake with its message and am beginning to understand my inner visions and dreams and new opportunities for healing which are opening for me. My inner feminine—now labeled a "friend"—is accompanying me and will continue to help me. I'm making progress. But I am not yet fully aware of this on a conscious level. I did not interpret these snake dreams and bring their messages to consciousness for several more years.

VARIOUS CONTRIBUTING FACTORS

Among the various theories as to causes of breast cancer is one suggesting that women who have spent their lives caring for and nurturing others and, perhaps, not looking out for their own needs, are likely candidates for breast cancer. Vernon Sylvest told me, "You need to focus on being relaxed and less concerned on making everyone around you happy. You need to reduce stress and your need to 'over-mother.' Then whatever you will do will work. You need to focus on being relaxed, on joy, on love, on gratitude every moment. All molecules will live blissfully. It takes discipline of the mind."

Years later I read Marilyn C. Barrick's *Dreams: Exploring the Secrets of Your Soul.* In this she discusses various alternative therapies, such as visualization, guided imagery, color and music therapy, energy medicine, emotional-release techniques and massage therapy. She states:

> Holistic doctors are consulted more and more by people looking for natural alternatives to drug therapy. . . . All of these approaches are ultimately ways of drawing upon our higher spiritual energy to correct the subtle energy flow into our mind, emotions and physical body. The bottom line is that when we exercise right spirit, right mind, right desiring and right action, we bring healing energy into our world.

> The power of a transformational experience can not be underestimated. Change comes from within, not from without, and the experience places the locus of control back within us, where we can recognize it as our own healing system being activated.
>
> — Drs. Michael Greenwood & Pete Nunn, *Paradox & Dreaming: Medicine, Mythology & Transformation*

OVER-MOTHERING

It took me years to realize that I was "over-mothering" people. I have been helped to understand this tendency through study of the Enneagram, a framework for understanding more about ourselves that goes back many centuries and is consistent with modern psychological theories, including those of Freud, Jung, and Horney. There are numerous books available on the subject for those interested in exploring the system. Richard Riso in the preface of his book, *Personality Types: Using the Enneagram for Self-Discovery,* states:

> The personality types of the Enneagram identify the chief features of our inner landscape—where the precipitous cliffs, arid deserts, and treacherous quicksands of the soul lie, as well as where the fertile oases, resourceful forests, and life-producing springs are within us. . . . [U]nderstood and used properly, the Enneagram is not merely a map of our states of personality but a map that points the way toward what lies beyond us, once we have transcended ourselves.

As I began the study of this system I found it very confusing and difficult to decide where I fit among the nine personality types. I gradually realized I fit in Type Two: The Helper. "Twos make it their business to solve everyone's problems." I simply wanted to help others, friends and family. But Riso states:

> Average Twos inevitably overextend themselves, helping too many people, sitting on too many committees, giving advice to too many friends, until they begin to feel burdened and physically worn out by their charity. Yet it is difficult for them not to be so involved, since that is how they maintain their sense of self.

Riso discusses the difference between Healthy Twos and Unhealthy Twos. The latter are seeking love through doing things for others, unconscious of such motives, sometimes being manipulative while trying to feel loved and cared for. They may unconsciously try another avenue, a physical illness. Then others will have to take care of them. The illnesses that result are those in which stress plays an important role.

Average Twos can become Healthy Twos by getting in touch with their feelings, including ones they would label negative feelings—anger and aggression. They can become aware of themselves as they really are, accepting negative feelings as well as positive ones. This doesn't mean that one should act on the negative feelings, just accept the fact one has them and perhaps express them in some non-harmful manner. When Twos unconditionally accept themselves as they do others, it is

> possible to give something deeper and more personal to others than they have ever done in the past. And when they are loved by others, it is all the more gratifying because others love the whole of them. Integrating Twos can rightly feel that they are no longer loved just for what they do for others, but for who they are.

Wanting to become fully conscious of the workings of my psyche, I began to question my motives. Could it be that I have had unconscious needs that I have attempted to satisfy through actions I considered purely altruistic?

In the late 1970s some doctors began to suspect a connection between how we think and feel and the strength of our immune system and that this connection can influence our ability to prevent or recover from certain diseases, including cancer. Internationally acclaimed psychologist Dr. Lydia Temoshok conducted a series of scientific studies which she describes in *The Type C Connection: The Behavioral Links to Cancer and Your Health*, co-authored with Henry Dreher. She describes the behavioral pattern, which she named "Type C," that she observed in the patients studied. One of the characteristics she found was "that these patients had always been completely devoted to pleasing their spouses, parents, siblings, friends, or coworkers. Their very identity seemed to depend wholly upon the reflected acceptance of those people significant in their lives." This sounds like what Richard Riso calls the "Unhealthy Twos." Dr. Temoshok explains further that "[b]ecause Type C behavior mainly influences our immune defenses, it stands to reason that Type C will have more impact on cancers that we can resist immunologically. Our immune defenses are better able to control some cancers than others. For example, the role of immune containment has been more well established in melanoma, colon cancer, and breast cancer."

These studies seem to validate Vernon Sylvest's instruction to be less concerned with making everyone around me happy. I should realize that my own needs are important. I need to nurture myself.

> I knew I had to learn to attend to *my* needs, not to act out of a requirement for other's approval or respect.
>
> — Barbara Marie Brewster, *Journey to Wholeness*

SELF-NURTURE

What does one do to nurture oneself? How does one really know this is what is needed? I found some answers in my dreams.

Wednesday morning, April 6, a week after beginning radiation treatments, I recalled several dreams. In one I was concerned about a woman who denied she had had a lumpectomy. This seemed to be telling me my unconscious had not yet accepted my illness. This dream was followed by another which may have been suggesting ways to nurture myself.

A Commode Morphs into a Spa Tub

I am observing scenes, observing a woman doing things, yet somehow I feel the things are happening to me. The woman needs the bathroom and is shown where one is. The seat is some sort of low ceramic bowl which she sits down upon.

The scene fades away, but later I am observing the woman again. The low bowl has become a large, low spa-type tub and has filled with water. The tub has become something very soft and the woman is lounging very comfortably, thoroughly enjoying the luxurious feeling of it all. I think this is great and am glad for her, thinking it is good for her to have this to enjoy.

The introductory and closing sentences show that my ego is becoming aware of other aspects of myself, represented by "the woman," and "I" am glad to discover ways to nurture myself. In dreams a bathroom often represents a place to gets things out of one's system, either eliminating waste products—things the body no longer needs and/or toxins—or expressing feelings and opinions. Inability—in waking life—to do this can lead to physical illness. The woman is being shown where to find a bathroom. Perhaps the radiation treatments are a means of getting rid of lingering, unwanted cells. On another level perhaps the dream is showing me a way to express myself.

The second part of the dream is intriguing. The ceramic bowl commode morphs into a soft, spa-type tub in which the woman can lounge and enjoy herself. This part is showing me a way to nurture myself; I should take opportunities such as one would find in a spa to pamper and nurture myself. This also brings to mind the idea that bathing can be considered a spiritual ritual. From ancient times to the present some form of symbolic bathing—immersion, pouring, or sprinkling—has been among humankind's rituals signifying cleansing, healing, and renewal coming from a divine, life-giving force. It can be a valuable way to regain harmony and balance in one's life. In their article in the August 2003 *Spirituality & Health,* Nadine Epstein and Rosita Arvigo suggest that "[s]piritual bathing can open the door to one's own inner guidance, uplifting the soul to foster a more reverent, peaceful state of mind. . . . [It] is intertwined with healing practices throughout the world and can benefit even those who do not hold any particular religious or spiritual beliefs. . . . [I]t incorporates two essential components: water and prayer."

For years I have enjoyed long, soaking tub baths, finding them very relaxing at the end of the day's activities. I have often been in a deep meditative state while there. I should add the missing ingredient—conscious prayer.

Additional dreams following my radiation treatments show that I still need to pay more attention to my own needs. On Sunday, May 15, 1994, eleven days after my last radiation treatment, I had this dream:

The Teacher Takes Care of My Kitten

I am going to school and it is an all-day session for several days in a row. I don't remember whether I stayed overnight. But I have taken a kitten with me to care for. I evidently am involved in my school work and am not paying attention to the kitten. I notice that the teacher has gotten the kitten and is putting it into a large covered-over pen made of cardboard. Also she is putting a litter pan in for the kitten. I hadn't thought of this need for the kitten during the day. I am very pleased the teacher has thought of this and is concerned for the kitten.

In one approach to working with dreams all people and animals in a dream may represent parts of the dreamer. Over the years I have had many dreams about kittens—adorable animals I have loved all my life. Soon after we married, "kitten" became the pet name Owen called me. Thus it was natural that I came to realize that a kitten in a dream could easily be a symbol for a part of myself. With this in mind, we can see that the above dream is saying that the ego part of me—the "I"—is not paying enough attention to the kitten part of me. But the teacher part of me is. "I" am pleased that at least one part of me is aware of my needs, and perhaps "I" will learn from my teacher how to take care of myself.

A year later I may be finally realizing the need to take care of myself. On April 25, 1995, I dreamed:

I Show My Mother a Kitten

I pick up a small kitten and need to care for it as if it were a special child. I may take it to show an older woman, maybe my mother.

On August 28, 1995, I dreamed:

I Need to Take Care of the Motherless Kitten

I'm trying to lead my pets, maybe to come home. One cat is entangled in a bush. Later I find strange cats in my yard. I bring one into the house to show someone else. It is just a tiny kitten. I comment that it is too young to be leaving its mother. I wonder how I can take care of it , but I think I need to, because I don't see its mother around anywhere.

There is a reference in the last two dreams to a mother. In the first of these two dreams I want to show my mother the kitten. In the latter, the kitten is without its mother and needs to be cared for. Dreams may have more than one level of meaning. On one level I may simply be wanting to show the kitten to my mother. But my biological mother died in 1966, therefore the reference is probably to the "mother" part of myself. Certainly the kitten part of myself needs mothering, nurturing by the maternal part. Since my mother is deceased, I need to do this for myself.

> Our immune system is only as strong as the dosage of self-love, self-acceptance, and self-care that we administer to ourselves daily.
>
> — Rusty Berkus,
> *Appearances,* cited in
> Barbara Marie Brewster,
> *Journey to Wholeness*

GRIEF

It is often stated that a serious illness might follow approximately two years after the loss of a loved one. This seems to fit my circumstances since the cancer was diagnosed at the end of December 1993, two years after my father died. But then I question this theory because I have read that breast cancer takes ten years to develop within one's body.

With my father's death on December 20,1991, I became a "grown orphan." Father survived my mother by twenty-five years. His continued presence during those years was very important to me. I had always felt very close to him and I realize I adopted many of his characteristics. I was thankful that our children were able to know their grandfather as they were growing up. He was a very energetic, active man all his life, up until about a month before his death at age ninety-six. I spent a large portion of that last month of his life sitting by his bedside.

Perhaps an even greater loss to my psyche was my mother's death in 1966. I was only thirty-two years old and our children were five and one years old. I find I'm still grieving over the loss of my mother. It hits me in waves of emotion. I have already mentioned such a time occurring at the time of my stepmother's funeral. I think of all the times missed relating to her as an adult. She would have been so interested in my most recent developments (dreamwork, spirituality, art) and in my interest in writing. She had many artistic talents. She had drawings skills, although she did not use them. Her main creative outlet was weaving. On her floor loom she wove table linens, bedspreads, and even material for a suit coat for my father. She did try her hand at writing, I remember, and I still have several of her manuscripts—one in particular, a story about artificial insemination, which was a relatively new idea when she was writing about it. She would have loved seeing her grandchildren grow up. They missed knowing her. She was a "nurturer extraordinaire." As has been discussed earlier, I have further grief work to do.

Another contributing factor might be stress. Vernon Sylvest said I needed to reduce stress. Sandra McLanahan thought the cancer was related to taking estrogen and to stress, in particular the loss of my father. She said deep sadness can affect the immune system.

STRESS

Stress can come in different forms. Sadness—grief—is stressful. Aggravations, perhaps beginning with small things that "bug" you, are stressful. My dream of not wanting to sleep in a bed full of fleas (discussed earlier) showed I felt an urgent need of getting away from things that were bugging me. Three years later a dream showed I was trying to get rid of any lingering bugs. This time I was clearing bugs—even dead bugs—from the floor of my closet.

Unacknowledged or repressed anger can certainly cause stress. Southern girls growing up in the first half of the twentieth century had it drilled into them that they should serve others and not express anger. Therefore we considered anger a negative feeling that we would not want to acknowledge having. Sandra McLanahan, when I saw her on February 8, suggested that I ask for a dream for information such as "what am I angry about?" I wasn't aware of any unexpressed anger, but I did try to incubate a dream as she suggested. I didn't get one at the time. But in reviewing earlier dreams I discovered one I had had eight months earlier. On Friday, June 11, 1993 before I had any hint that I might have breast cancer, I had a dream which seems to be calling my attention to one factor that possibly contributed towards my getting cancer.

I Fear the Fire Will Spread Beyond the Contained Area

I am in the home of someone like the college president's wife—in a room with a fireplace—or some kind of fire burning area. I am concerned about the fire because it looks to me as if it is extending beyond the desired area and about to ignite rugs or something right beyond the edge of the fire. I try to tactfully point this out to the woman but she doesn't want to hear it or accept the idea that there is a problem.

Dream analyst Jeremy Taylor suggests rewriting the dream to help us understand it. In front of each verb add "I am" and after nouns add "part of me." Thus the above dream might read:

> *I am in the home part of me of someone like the college president's wife part of me in a room part of me with a fireplace part of me, or some kind of fire burning area part of me. I am concerned about the fire part of me because it looks to me as if I am extending beyond the desired area part of me (which contains the fire) and I am about to ignite the rugs part of me or something right beyond the edge of the fire part of me. I am trying to tactfully point this out to the woman part of me but she doesn't want to hear it or accept the idea that there is a problem part of me.*

When we first read this rewritten dream it may sound strange and stilted. But let's take a closer look at it. Since most of the verbs in the dream already say "I am," only a few needed a slight alteration. Let's consider in detail the various nouns that have been altered. This actually can help us understand the symbols in the dream. Home became "home part of me"; room became "room part of me"; fireplace became "fireplace part of me." It is generally thought that a house in a dream stands for oneself and the rooms of the house represent various aspects of one's body or personality. The first revised sentence in the dream seems to spell this out. Next, consider what the fireplace and fire parts represent. Fireplace is considered a place of warmth and nurturing. Fire can be a symbol of positive zeal or purification and transformation or it can be destructive anger or passion or any strong emotion burning out of control. Which it is depends on the context of the dream. In this dream it might be considered destructive since I state it is extending beyond the desired area. What does a rug stand for? Perhaps the part of one that gets walked on and thus is used or abused.

My mother was a college president's wife. Thus the dream is discussing that part of me that is like my mother. And that part does not want to hear or accept the idea that there is a problem. Notice also that I—the ego part of me—even felt it necessary to be "tactful" while pointing out the problem to my mother and I am concerned that the fire will spread beyond the acceptable contained area. In considering this dream I asked myself if my mother was afraid of expressing anger, fearing it would get out of control or be unacceptable. Have I adopted the same beliefs? Would it be so bad for the rug to get burned, or would the opposite be true? In other words, does that part of me that gets abused, walked on, need to go? Do I need to express my anger rather than contain it?

The "woman" part of me thus can represent a specific part of myself; it can also represent "woman" in general. This can bring up the whole issue of cultural indoctrinations and women's rights. I have already mentioned that girls growing up in the first half of the twentieth century had it drilled into them to serve others and not express anger; we should think it not a problem when we contain it. Now I am very conscious that I followed this approach. I feared I would make the other person feel bad if I expressed my anger. In fact, I often would not even realize I was angry since I had buried these feelings, pushed them out of my awareness. In the dream, my mother didn't want to hear about or acknowledge a problem. But this is exactly why I had the dream. It is telling me to pay attention. There is something I need to be aware of and do something about. I need to realize that expressing my anger can be beneficial to me. Keeping such feelings bottled up inside might lead to health problems. Dr. Temoshok states in her book that "[m]ind-body researchers have found that a life-long tendency to repress anger and other negative emotions may be one factor that gradually weakens our biological defense again cancer."

> It appears that suppression of grief and suppression of anger, in particular, is associated with an increased incidence of breast cancer in women.
>
> — Candace Pert, Ph.D., cited by Bill Moyers, *Healing and the Mind*

At several conferences I have been privileged to hear a well-known workshop leader in the fields of psychology and psychoneuroimmunology and therapist in private practice, Paula M. Reeves. She states: "When you don't know or care what matters most to you, that then becomes the matter with you." Dreams give us a chance to check in and see what is "mattering" to us.

Rachel Naomi Remen points out in *My Grandfather's Blessings* the importance and value of coming to know oneself and what really matters. She says that many people with cancer have told her

> that they have not spoken their truth to others for years out of fear of rejection or some other form of loss or because they find themselves living or working among people who see things differently than they do. They have become invisible in order to survive or maintain the status quo. But when we do not live coherently with ourselves, something begins to erode in us. We may survive, but we will never be whole or fully alive. . . . Becoming separated from our authentic values may weaken us. This may be why, when people's lives are challenged by significant illness and they instinctively begin to gather their strength, their values are often among the first things that change. . . . Sometimes it takes a wake-up call like cancer to bring us back to ourselves. The crisis of illness may shake us free of the life that we have created and allow us to begin a return to the life that is our own.

I know that in my own case sometimes I felt I should not express anger and differing opinions. I believe that this is what the fourth dream of the "initial dream series" was trying to point out to me.

I Go into the Men's Room

> *4. At one point I need the bathroom. I find one and go in. While in there I realize I have gone in the men's room. I don't want to be found in there and I don't want anyone to know I have gone in the wrong place. I don't think anyone knows or realizes what has happened.*

As I have stated earlier, a bathroom can represent a place to express feelings and opinions, as well as get rids of toxic wastes. In this dream I find such a place, but I seem to fear there might be trouble if other people learn I was in the men's room, not the women's room. What is the difference symbolically? Since masculine attributes within one's personality are considered much more assertive than the feminine, perhaps my using the men's room might suggest I'm being more assertive than others might think proper for a female. In the dream I don't want others to know that's where I have been. This seems to point out my hesitancy to assert myself, at least in a visible way, even though this is what I need to do. I've held back from expressing anger and differing opinions because I thought such expressions would displease the other person, would upset them too much. I did this with good intentions, thinking I was serving the well-being of the other person. This idea was part of my upbringing as a girl during the 1930s and 1940s. But I learned, as already mentioned, I needed to think of my own needs more. Many women with breast cancer learn this. When we then begin to make changes within relationships, other people in our lives feel thrown off balance. Why aren't things continuing the way they always have been going? Some friendships may dissolve. Some marriages break up. It is hard to redefine relationships. It takes sincere efforts at loving communication and understanding to successfully shift one's *modus operandi*—one's way of interacting with other people.

I have come to realize a need for "my own space," time and a place for my own activities and time away from anyone else. I am not abandoning or rejecting other people, I simply need this for myself. On June 24, 1995, I dreamed:

I Need Peace and Quiet

I am in the house of my family (parents, brother, cousin, etc.). Much activity is going on. People are coming and going. I'm in the midst of all the activity, trying to help, organize, straighten out matters, etc. There are several main ground level rooms, where all the activity is going on. I'm pleased when the rooms are cleared of people and there is peace and quiet. I feel that when this happens, I can accomplish some things, attend to business which needs to be done. But fairly quickly people come back in and things become hectic and it's hard to do whatever work it is I need to do.

This dream is fairly straightforward, saying I need peace and quiet away from other people and the hustle and bustle of activities in order to accomplish what needs to be done. My life in the dream seems to be centered around activities involving parents, brother, and extended family. It shows that at this point I'm still operating from the standpoint of my upbringing (I am in the house of my family and am doing their business). This dream came after the kitten dreams mentioned above. Perhaps the dreammaker is hoping a different metaphor will make me pay attention to the need to do more for myself. I evidently have not come to terms with this issue, so the dreams keep reminding me.

My inner self continued to wrestle with the issue of needing my own space. Six years after this last mentioned dream and over seven years after completing treatments, on August 23, 2001, I had this dream:

I Lament Our Crowded Living Conditions

I'm living in some communal building where several people have to share the same space. It's very crowded and we lack privacy. On one occasion, I'm talking with another woman. We are lamenting our situation, saying we hope we'll be able to have our own rooms some day. She says it's not like we were in New York. She can understand crowding there. There is no room to spread out, just up, there. Here we have space. We ought not to have to live in such a crowded situation.

This dream speaks on one level to my own individual needs. The other women can represent the multiple feminine aspects of myself that desire more space. They can also represent women in general, thus the dream can be speaking on an archetypal level for the needs of all women.

A few months later, December 18, 2001, this dream:

I Search for My Assigned Space

I'm wandering through the hallway of a public building. I do not remember, in recall, where I am. I seem to be searching for a place to sit, or perhaps even to spend the night. This is not clear. It seems I have been assigned a place. I look past the door to my left, into what looks like a train compartment. I think this is my assigned space. I see an elderly man seated on one side. I decide to look further. When I look through the next doorway, I see a much larger space which looks like a large hospital room. I watch as a hospital bed or gurney is rolled from my right towards the empty area to the left. I back out of there; I don't want to stay there. I may look farther, but end up coming back to my assigned space which looks slightly different when I return. The man has moved, but I don't remember any more.

In this one I'm walking down a hallway (a place of transition), searching for a place to sit or spend the night, but it is an assigned place in a public building. Could it be saying I'm looking for my assigned role in life? Since it is a public building and the particular space looks like a train compartment and a train is a means of transportation for the masses, one might think this refers to the culturally assigned role for me—as an individual, and maybe in particular, as a woman. When I find the assigned place I'm not pleased with what I see. It is already occupied by an elderly man. Evidently I don't want to share a space. Deciding to look farther, I look through another doorway into what looks like a hospital room. I don't want to stay there. That's good; I don't want to be ill. I'll do whatever is necessary to avoid such a place, even going back to the assigned space. Maybe it won't be as much of a problem as I originally thought; the elderly man could be my inner "wise old man." The space "looks slightly different when I return." Maybe it's because I'm looking at things differently. "The man has moved." I had assumed this meant he left, but maybe he didn't. Maybe he's just sitting in a different spot. Perhaps I'm meant to occupy a place with him, perhaps we both have wisdom we can share with each other and with the masses.

There is another aspect to the need for one's own space. This has to do with defining one's space and is a way of setting boundaries. Physical boundaries can help define psychological boundaries. At times we can be so close (psychologically and emotionally) to someone that we feel bombarded by vibrations from this person. Modern science recognizes the fact that we send out "psychic vibrations" that can extend many feet in what is termed a "vibrational field." There are times when we need to put space between ourselves and someone else to help us disconnect from the other person's concerns in order not to feel overwhelmed. We sometimes refer to our problems as our "baggage." We don't want to carry around someone else's "stuff"; our own issues and problems fill up our suitcase. In May of 2002 I had a dream that uses the idea of baggage as its metaphor.

I Want Only My Things in My Suitcase

I am standing by as Owen is packing his suitcase for a trip he is to make by himself. He is taking his clothing out of my suitcase to put in his own suitcase. Perhaps we have just returned from a trip together during which we shared the one suitcase—mine. As he finishes up, I ask him if he wants the several shirts—long sleeve "dress" shirts—which remain in my suitcase. He seems to have forgotten they are there and asks what ones I mean. I say the ones still in my suitcase. He says, No, he doesn't need them for this trip. I want the shirts out of my suitcase, for I'm to be making my own trip and want all the space in my suitcase for my things.

This dream states that my husband and I have been on a trip together during which we shared one suitcase. But we are about to make separate trips. I believe the dreammaker is pointing out the fact that we have shared much on our life's journey together. But we also have separate journeys to make, our own pursuits to follow, our own quests to undertake. For this separate journey I wish to carry only my own stuff. This desire does not lessen my interest in what he is undertaking or my love and concern for him. It shows an acknowledgment of my own needs.

Feelings of being bombarded by other people's vibrations can be present even when you do not know the other people. I believe this is what makes me prefer a table in the corner or along the side of the room in restaurants. I feel very uncomfortable out in the middle where the chatter of conversations from surrounding tables seems to be overwhelming. This is what made me need to retreat by myself into an adjoining room during a family gathering for the funeral of Owen's uncle.

There is another way we may be carrying other people's baggage. Our suitcases may be filled with a set of beliefs or patterns of behavior that belonged to our parents and other authority figures from our childhood. I know we need to have guidelines as we are growing up, but we also need to be able to decide for ourselves as we mature which of beliefs seem right for us. However, it sometimes takes us many years to break free from some of these early indoctrinations. Our need and desire to do so may appear in our dreams in scenes of being imprisoned and trying to find a way to escape. Many of my earliest remembered dreams in the early 1970s have this theme. At the time I was in my late thirties and my children were in elementary and junior high schools. On Thursday, August 17, 1972, I had a very traumatic dream.

I Fear Animals and Humans Outside Our Tower Prison

Our family is imprisoned in a strange tower home surrounded by a fence and near an ocean. At first we are allowed outside for periods of time, but we always have to come back in. At times we have to hurry in to escape pursuit by fierce animals such as wild boars and wolves. We know we are being plotted against by an enemy, humans who control the wild beasts too. We feel it is just a matter of time before things will go from bad to worse. On one occasion whole flocks of birds (perhaps gulls or something similar) are out in front near the ocean and they stalk nearer and nearer the house or tower devouring something off the ground. At times we have to climb the fence to get in to safety before being caught. Sometimes the wolves or something similar will lie in wait outside the windows of the tower. I try to keep my son back from the windows as protection.

In this dream my family and I are imprisoned in a tower home surrounded by a fence. An "ivory tower" suggests to me an institution of learning, which seems applicable since we were living on a college campus and I also grew up on a college campus. In the dream this setting is confining. Confinement in dreams can represent a set of beliefs or patterns of behavior that inhibit one's personal development. My beliefs at the time probably came from at least three different sources: first from my parents who impressed upon me a preferred pattern of behavior and set of beliefs, second from teachers and other "authority figures" on both social and religious matters, and third from the present college community with its own set of expectations for one's behavior and activities.

It's interesting to note the dream states that "we are allowed outside for periods of time, but we always have to come back in." I apparently *want* to come back in; I seem to be more fearful of beasts and birds outside the enclosure and the humans who control them than I am of the confinement. Tony Crisp, in *Dream Dictionary*, describes an enclosure in dreams as "the defenses we use, such as pride, beliefs, anger, to protect ourselves from deeply feeling the impact of the world, relationship, love, anxiety, or pain. These are often felt as traps or restraints, even though they are parts of our personality." It seems to me that there is a double trap in this dream. We are imprisoned in the tower, but I feel threatened by the beasts and the birds that are outside the enclosure. Wolves are noble creatures, but they can represent traits which are mysterious, crafty, and deceptive. Wild beasts can represent emotional aspects or animal instincts which are uncontrolled and unpredictable. Evidently the beliefs that were instilled in me as I was growing up left me fearful of what I found in the outside world, and at the time of this dream, I felt overwhelmed by the situation; I felt it was just a matter of time before things would go from bad to worse. This dream illustrates how "baggage" from my early years had become extremely stressful, and I was not conscious of this fact.

Twenty-three years later, a year after my diagnosis, I was still dreaming of being in prison. But it is encouraging to see that I am, by this time, actively trying to escape. On Sunday, January 22, 1995, this was the story.

Trying to Escape an Institution

I am a prisoner of some group and am trying to escape. I'm not in a cell or confined in that way, maybe just confined in a building or institution. I go up to someone, or two, seated at a table and ask if I can use some paper they have. I'm not sure if there is already something on the paper, maybe a painting. I act as if I want to draw or paint on it, so that my "captors," if they are watching, will not realize what I'm really doing. I want to write an appeal for help. I turn to a page farther in a stack, or in a book, and write: "Please help me escape. I'm being held prisoner" or something kin to this. I'm not aware of any immediate response or help.

> *Later I'm still trying to figure out how to get away and out of the building. There is a last door to go out. I devise a method I think might work. I watch some woman who is leaving go to the exit area and she throws her keys—or something—over onto a counter at a place to the side near the entrance. This is evidently what is done when you leave the building. I decide that maybe if I do the same thing—acting very natural as I do this—no one will suspect anything wrong and I'll be able to leave. I do this—"the routine"—while the woman I appealed to for help is there. In fact the woman I observed is the same woman. Maybe she thought of this as a way of showing me how I can escape. She watches "with a knowing eye" and saying nothing as I toss the keys onto the counter. I either wake up or the dream shifts at this point.*

"I'm not in a cell or confined in that way, maybe just confined in a building or institution." After secretly appealing for help in escaping, some woman shows me how I might fool the authorities and make my escape. But I wake up before I escape.

George R. Slater suggests in *Bringing Dreams to Life* that "(i)mages of public buildings, such as institutional, governmental or business buildings, malls, and apartment buildings, inasmuch as they are impersonal, may refer to being trapped in collective thinking, where the individual is submerged by the institution. Inasmuch as they are manmade, they may refer to structures of a person's own life experience that have been socially imposed." So this dream echoes the ideas of the one many years ago. But this time, with the help of my inner feminine, I'm trying to leave a confining situation, to break away from constricting thoughts and beliefs, to generate—to call into existence—my own set of beliefs, to allow my own individuality to blossom. This dream occurred eight months before the dream of the bed full of fleas in which I express the urgent need to move to a new place. As I stated in the earlier discussion of that dream, I was needing to get away from old assumptions and expectations of what was important in my life and how I should behave. We have here a good example of more than one dream trying, from different approaches, to get the same idea across to the dreamer. At this time, my conscious mind was very much focused on the desire to move to Lake Monticello. We had purchased our lot there, but had not decided when we would build and move. Also months before this dream Drs. McLanahan and Sylvest had been telling me to nurture myself. I was wanting to do just this. The following dream from Saturday, January 13, 1996, shows I am making progress.

I Obey Authorities Against My Mother's Advice

I have found a small kitten who has been mistreated, abused, looks "beat up." I decide to care for it. For some reason which is not clear in my remembering, I'm supposed to report finding the kitten to some "authority." Someone with me (maybe my mother) advises me not to report my discovery. I insist that I should and then make a phone call to do so. The "authority" tells me that I will be fined. Why, I don't know. The person with me reminds me that she had advised me I shouldn't make the report; maybe somehow she knew this would happen. I tell the authority that fining me doesn't make sense. I've done nothing wrong. In fact, I'm trying to help the kitten by bringing it home and taking care of it, so it is very unfair to fine me. The person finally tells me she will just give me a "ticket." I won't have to pay out any money for a fine. This is a warning to not repeat my offense. Why this is a problem—in the dream, and in thinking about it, is a mystery to me.

In this dream we see the dreammaker using the kitten symbol again. Remember, too, that dreams exaggerate to make a point. I have found a "mistreated" kitten and intend to care for it. The strangest part is the requirement to report my find to "authorities," who then intend to penalize me with a "fine." Someone, maybe my mother—the nurturing part of me—advises me not to call the authorities, but I'm not able to go against my training to obey authorities, so I do call. The threat of a fine does seem very unfair since all I'm wanting to do is to take care of the kitten. The person in authority does give in to my plea, will just give me a ticket, but warns me to obey in the future. I believe this dream is trying to point out the need for me to decide for myself what is right. The "authority" figure in the dream represents external authorities who have established rules, who tell people including me what we must do. There are times when external rules are needed. But there are also times when such rules do not "make sense," seem unfair, and will produce undesirable, unhealthy results. In my dream, following the external authority's rule would result in depriving an animal of safety and nurture. In such circumstances we need to depend on our own judgment, our internal authority, to guide our behavior. These are times when we need to go beyond the boundaries we learned as children. Since we know from prior discussion that the animal—the kitten—represents me, the dream is saying this is what I need to do.

In 1998 and 1999 I attended the Institute for the Enhancement of Dreamwork. We met for a weekend every three months to be instructed by leading Jungian dreamworkers on various aspects of dreamwork. We also gained experience in working with groups on our own dreams. Before one of the last sessions, our assignment was to review our dreams and life events of the past eighteen months. Then, one assignment during that weekend, Sunday, July 25, 1999, was to "pull together" thoughts from our review in some expressive form. Observing how many of my dreams were suggesting the need for me to go beyond boundaries set by early "authorities' in my life, I decided to draw a mandala showing energies extending themselves beyond the circular boundary of the mandala. Although I consciously extended colors beyond the circle, the particular colors used and their placement evolved intuitively. Someone recently pointed out to me the similarity of this mandala to the "Emotions" painting created the weekend I awaited the diagnosis. Yes, they both seem to show a volcanic eruption, a boiling up of emotions and/or energies. The difference can be seen in the colors present or missing. This mandala has all the primary and secondary colors, which suggests wholeness. I used a rainbow of colors which in themselves suggest a full range of energies present within my body and psyche, available to help me go beyond the early boundaries in many new directions. In "Emotions" the "primary" blue—the color of nurturing, peace, and calmness—and green—the color of harmony and healing—are missing. This mandala, which I have entitled *Breaking Through Boundaries,* is included on page 100.

Two months after drawing this mandala, on Tuesday, September

21, 1999, I had the following dream.

No Longer Will the Woman Hide from Authorities

Some female that I know is being sought by "authorities." I do not know the reason, but she seeks a place to hide. Several of us help her. She hides in some small container. I forget what, but it is something that the authorities would not suspect as a hiding place. Those in pursuit come by, look around, and do not find her. We are standing around watching, but do not reveal we know where she is. I assume they leave. Later she decides to come out of hiding—that she will hide no longer—even if it means she'll be discovered.

Although we are not told why the woman is hiding from the authorities, we might assume that she has done something in defiance of their rules. It is likely she has decided for herself what action or path in life is right for her. This, of course, represents a part of myself that is doing just this. However, it appears that in the beginning of the dream I'm still unsure of myself and feel the need to hide from these authority figures. The most encouraging part happens when the woman in the dream—this part of me—decides she will hide no longer; she will acknowledge her position to the authorities, and thus to the world. It appears that I am beginning to go beyond earlier confining boundaries and to make new boundaries based on my own intuitive guides as to what is right for me.

With this last series of dreams we have seen how there are two aspects to establishing boundaries. In one, we need to set boundaries to reserve our own space. In the other, we need to expand or break through confining boundaries prescribed at an earlier time.

So far I've discussed psychological factors which might lead to physical problems. We also need to consider actual physical circumstances and activities.

> [T]he energy required to suppress unwanted feelings has to go somewhere, and it usually goes into the body. . . . Through transforming our fundamental outlook, the energy which is locked up in chronic tension patterns can be released, and healing can occur in all dimensions of our being.
>
> — Drs. Michael Greenwood & Pete Nunn, *Paradox & Dreaming: Medicine, Mythology & Transformation*

HORMONE REPLACEMENT THERAPY

Sandra McLanahan thought one of the factors contributing to having breast cancer was taking estrogen in Hormone Replacement Therapy. Whenever I questioned other doctors about this possibility, most of them said "no way." The surgeon whom I consulted for a second opinion before the lumpectomy sensed my concern about having taken Premarin. He stated that it would not have given me the cancer. When I mentioned that one doctor thought it might have contributed, he said he'd like to be shown the proof. My radiologist thought the estrogen might have stimulated some normal glandular changes that might have masked the situation. The cancer might have been seen sooner otherwise, but he didn't think it would make any difference. He stated, "There is no evidence that estrogen causes breast cancer."

My own intuition agreed with Sandra McLanahan. I was glad I had decided to taper off and quit taking the HRT when I did. Then immediately after my diagnosis my gynecologist announced I should not take any more hormones. I reminded her that I was already tapering off. In fact, I had only a fraction of a pill left and I would not take this.

In 1998, needing to find a gynecologist in Charlottesville (my former one was in Richmond), I consulted someone who had been recommended as one of the top ten cancer specialists in the country. Though very friendly, he was an "old-school" M.D. who didn't think much of some alternative options. He announced that he didn't think HRT had anything to do with my getting breast cancer. He said the kind I had was very unusual and he had never seen any evidence that it would be caused by estrogens. To counter some post-menopausal symptoms, he recommended the use of a vaginal ring (Estring) which releases estrogens locally into the vagina. He said he thought it perfectly safe to use. I asked if he had any written information on it that I could have. He found two pamphlets which he said he had not read and therefore couldn't discuss what they said. I came home feeling frustrated and confused. After getting home, I read the pamphlets. They advised *against using* the Estring if you have had breast cancer! I definitely did not want to use it.

In recent years studies have been made that show results validating Sandra McLanahan's opinion. A large clinical trial of HRT in post-menopausal women was undertaken by the Women's Health Initiative. This was halted early during the summer of 2002 when it showed an increased incidence of breast cancer and heart disease. According to the *New York Times* News Service as cited in the *Richmond Times-Dispatch* on June 25, 2003, researchers reported in the *Journal of the American Medical Association* new findings from this study. "[T]he combination of hormones used in a common type of therapy makes tumors harder to detect, leading to dangerous delays in diagnosis. . . . Women who take the combination are also more likely to have changes in their breast tissue that lead to abnormal mammograms, problems that can show up during the first year of hormone use. . . . [These] findings raise questions about the safety of even short term use." Even though many of the abnormalities turn out to be harmless, further tests—including biopsies—are usually needed, causing anxieties and possibly involving risks. In December 2002 the National Institute of Environmental Health listed an entire class of steroidal estrogens in the category of greatest hazard. New information concerning the dangers of estrogen therapies are being announced with increasing regularity. My early concerns regarding such dangers have been validated. Recent theories that a natural (bio-identical) hormone—a custom product that supplies one's body with the same hormones it is used to seeing—can be used without the side effects associated with synthetic HRT may offer an alternative. But personally I do not feel comfortable with this idea and do not want any dangerous potential to be a part of my scenario.

DIET AND EXERCISE

> The best diet for healing from and preventing breast cancer is a whole foods diet consisting largely of unprocessed, unrefined whole grains and a wide variety of organic vegetables. This diet is mineral- and vitamin-rich, naturally low-fat, low-protein, high-fiber and non-dairy.
>
> — Barbara Joseph,
> *My Healing from Breast Cancer*

I gained a lot of weight in the years leading up to my cancer diagnosis. Perhaps this contributed to my risk of cancer. After following the strict diet and exercise program prescribed by Sandra McLanahan, I lost a large amount of weight—a big part of the forty-four pounds I lost in a period of eight months ending after my diagnosis. The mammogram taken six months after the suspicious one showed the spot had not increased in size during the intervening time. I felt I had been doing something right.

To answer the question "Can diet, nutrition and exercise influence one's breast cancer risk?" the National Cancer Institute states in *Everyone's Guide to Cancer Therapy*: "Fat stores estrogen (some breast cancers are estrogen-dependent), so the more fit and trim we are, the better our health." Therefore it was, and still is, very important for me to watch my diet and to keep my weight down.

In my reading I came across some very convincing scientific information in Jane A. Plant's book, *Your Life in Your Hands: Understanding, Preventing, and Overcoming Breast Cancer.* Plant, one of Britain's most outstanding scientists and the 1999 recipient of Britain's most prestigious science honor—the Lord Lloyd of Kilgerran Prize—contracted breast cancer in 1987 and had five recurrences. After orthodox medicine gave up and told her she had only three months to live, she set out to find a way to survive. Using her extensive scientific training and knowledge, she became convinced there was a causal link between consumption of dairy products and breast cancer. Within days of eliminating all dairy products from her diet, the large "secondary" tumor comprising cancer cells in the lymph nodes of her neck started to shrink. Six weeks later the lump was no longer there.

The detailed evidence she gives in her book strongly "suggests that consuming dairy products (milk and meat [beef from dairy cattle]), including low-fat products such as yogurt, does indeed increase the risk of breast and prostate cancer in exposed populations." She also discovered that she was not the first person to advise against the use of dairy products. Dr. R. M. Kradjian, M.D., Chief of the Breast Surgery Division of General Surgery at the Seton Medical Center, in Daly City, California, did so in his book *Save Yourself from Breast Cancer.* Plant gives a clear statement of the scientific principles behind her discovery. She also includes detailed suggestions of ways to eliminate or reduce one's consumption of suspected cancer-causing agents and to replace them with healthy alternatives.

I am, of course, not in a position to fully evaluate Plant's experience and proposal. It does seem to be, however, the sort of recommendation that calls for further investigation.

I know that I need to do much more in the area of aerobic exercise. I have been sporadic in my efforts through the years. I have never been the athletic type person, but there are various avenues for getting the much needed and beneficial exercise. Walking is one of the best. Participation in a class or an individual program at a local fitness center are other possibilities. Recreational dancing would also be helpful.

It seems clear to me now that I, as an individual, need to do everything possible on many fronts to discourage any likelihood of a recurrence of cancer. In July of 1999 I had a dream which suggests I can do this.

I Will Accept the Role of Doctor

I'm attending a gathering where a serious discussion of the needs of the community is being held. It is decided that someone needs to be appointed to the role of "doctor." They begin considering who should be asked to accept this role. After some consideration some woman speaks up, turning to me asks, "How about you? Do you think you would consider doing this?"

If I were a young person starting to consider what should be my life work, I would think the dream is asking "Do you want to be a doctor?" But at age sixty-five, I hardly would consider beginning major medical training. The dream continues:

> *I respond that perhaps I would. I sense that some in the group are puzzled, perhaps amazed that I would consider myself able to do this. As I'm speaking, possible ideas begin to form in my mind. I think to myself that my Reiki [a kind of Therapeutic Touch] ability is a form of administering healing. I almost say this out loud, but then I decide it wiser not to. I also think I would be able to listen to the concerns of young teenage girls and perhaps could inspire them in various ways. I look around at several standing nearby and I begin to hum a tune with a "catchy" rhythm. First one and then another of the girls begin to join in the singing and to let their bodies sway in time to the tune. I spontaneously decide to lead them in a dance line, and motion for them to follow me. Gradually the whole group joins in and I lead a dancing line around an adjoining field. I think to myself that this kind of activity is "healing" and would be beneficial as a form of exercise. It would be good for me to encourage this by example and my own enthusiasm. This will inspire without their even being aware of what it is doing for them. They will consider it a fun activity that they enjoy doing. I ponder to myself whom I would be able to help this way. I answer my own question with the words "inner city people who do not have access to help."*

Is this saying I want to help the needy by actually becoming an "inner city" doctor? Not likely. Since I am a woman past retirement age, who survived a serious illness five years prior to this dream, what could this mean? I have been trained in the healing practice of Reiki and have considered putting this ability to use more publicly. But in the dream I decide it "wiser not to. . . say this out loud," and in waking life I decided against doing Reiki as a profession.

In one approach to dreamwork, everything in a dream represents a part of oneself. So a "community" could be everything that makes up the dreamer, all aspects of the person, one's personality, health, abilities, fears, anxieties, hopes, etc. The phrase "inner city people" supports this idea, perhaps meaning my inner parts, physical, mental and spiritual.

I think I am acknowledging to a part of myself that I can be my own healing force. Other parts may wonder whether this is possible. I can use my Reiki healing ability on myself. I can do various things to inspire and encourage the still young part of myself. To promote continued good health, I realize I need exercise. Many forms of exercise have never appealed to me, even when I was young. But singing and dancing to beautiful music have always been fun. As a young child I danced around the house to the tune of Strauss waltzes and other music played on our old-time Victrola. Doing this now would be very beneficial and healing.

> Exercise is also essential nourishment for the body. A balance of exercise with adequate rest is the goal. . . . Women who are physically active have lower cancer rates, better immune system function and enjoy many other overall health benefits.
>
> — Barbara Joseph,
> *My Healing from Breast Cancer*

Since we do not know with any certainty the causes of cancer, the best we can do is listen to advice from authorities who have investigated the question and to the inner guidance—the healing insights—of our own dreams. One of the very helpful resources now available is the McLanahans' *Surgery and Its Alternatives,* which discusses not only surgery, but also preventive measures and complementary treatments of numerous diseases and disorders. Once we have gathered as much information as possible, we should follow our own intuitive directives while making decisions about treatments and prevention of a recurrence. In my own experience I received additional valuable guidance through my dreams.

8

Listening to Inner Wisdom

By learning to contact, listen to, and act on our intuition, we can directly connect to the higher power of the universe and allow it to become our guiding force.
— Shakti Gawain

There is an amazing well of wisdom and guidance that may be found deep within us, in an area that cannot be seen with the physical eye. Carl Jung labeled it the Self (with the capital S). As Murray Stein explains in *Jung's Map of the Soul,* it ". . . is transcendent, which means that it is not defined by or contained within the psychic realm but rather lies beyond it and, in an important sense, defines it." It may be reached through prayer, meditation, and listening to our dreams, but this may take many years.

What is doubly amazing is that this part which I have frequently referred to as the dreammaker seems to have knowledge of possible occurrences long before we are aware of them in waking life. Such dreams in which symptoms of illness seem to appear prior to their arrival in waking life are called "prodromic," which Patricia Garfield tells us in *Creative Dreaming* comes "from the Greek word *prodromos,* meaning 'running before.'" While we are more familiar with the term "precognitive" relating to knowledge of an event or state not yet experienced, the word "prodromic" relates specifically to symptoms of disease. By recording and working with our dreams we can come to know what symbols represent our physical conditions, making it possible for us to take prompt preventive or corrective measures. The problem is most of us don't know enough in advance of a diagnosis to make this possible.

In looking back over my dreams beginning two years before my diagnosis, I discovered several dreams that possibly were trying to warn me. They seem to be examples of my unconscious knowing what was going on within my body long before the knowledge came into consciousness.

One dream of March 4, 1992, recounted:

> ***Large Insects Are Damaging Our Room***
>
> *Owen and I are living in a dorm room at some institution. We awake early morning to discover a terrible problem in our room. There are many—perhaps hundreds—of insects I'll call bees, but they are much larger and a different shape from bees, drilling holes in the wall behind our bed and eating big sections out of the top of the furniture, in particular, an antique dresser. Somehow—as a result of the holes in the walls—water is dripping down the walls. It is a mess and is very threatening. I go seeking help, then return to find Owen has already pulled many of our belongings including some furniture out into the hall. . . . Some things have also been stacked in the room next door. I go into this room to get something I need and find that the person or persons there are still in bed, maybe even still unaware of what is going on. . . . Before I returned to the room I had stopped in a girl's room at the far corner of the building. I noticed that there were some of the terrible bees in her room. I tried to tell her how terrible our situation is. We have so much more and they are doing such terrible things. I feel she could get rid of them before they do any damage if she only would. They have not begun to do damage there yet.*

A house or building can represent a person's body. In this dream some terrible insects are eating away at the walls of the room and furniture within the room. My first thoughts were that large bees don't seem to be enough like cancer cells to represent them. But later, upon rereading this dream, another possibility jumped into my head. Perhaps an aha! When I came to the part "there were some terrible bees in her (the girl's) room" I thought the "bees" can stand for "breasts" as well as the cancer cells. The dreammaker likes to use puns, euphemisms, metaphors, and symbols. Of course,

I don't think breasts are terrible. But, in one sense, they might be considered "terrible" if they were cancerous. The large size of the insects in the beginning of the dream may be the dreammaker's exaggeration to call attention to the problem. The fact that bees are in more than one place is another way of emphasizing the problem. The dream stated in no uncertain terms: "It is a mess and is very threatening." The person or persons in the room next door are "still unaware of what is going on." They and the girl in the far corner room can be multi-representations of myself. I am trying to warn myself of the terrible danger. "I feel she could get rid of them [the bees—the cancer cells] before they do any damage if she only would. They have not begun to do damage there yet." If I had only been able to recognize these signs in my dream at that time, perhaps I could have stopped the progress of the illness.

Our unconscious will keep trying to get a message across to us; if one way doesn't work, it tries a different one. We dream variations of the same theme until we consciously see what it is saying. Here again are examples of a kitten being used as the symbol for myself in an attempt to make me pay attention.

On March 22, 1992, I dreamed:

My Kitten's Strange Growth Needs to Be Cut Off

I have a pet cat that I love. I discover it has a branching (shrub-like) growth coming out of its body's underside. I hunt for the kitten to get it so I can cut off this growth. I find the kitten under a sideboard, pick it up and hold it lovingly.

The image of the "branching, shrub-like growth" is powerful. The dreammaker is trying to make the image more realistic.

On April 10, 1992 I dreamed:

A Growth on My Neck Needs to Be Removed

I have a strange growth coming out from the back side of the neck on the right side. I evidently had not done anything about it and it is continuing to grow. Later I become concerned because it is getting very large . . . . I decide something will have to be done. I will have it removed.

Obviously, the location of the growth is not in the "correct" position for breast cancer. Maybe the dreammaker moved the problem to a different location to make it more visible.

A different symbol was used in the following dream on April 22, 1992:

I Worry about Dangerous Growths in Our House

My family is living in a certain "official" house because of our job. There are people to help when we entertain. But I become very concerned with certain conditions in the house which I feel are dirty, unhealthy, and unsafe. The main thing I remember is the floor and its covering in the main large living room. It is covered with a heavy layer of white "dust" or moldy growth. There are actually plant-like growths coming up which can be grasped and pulled up. I feel that the white covering is very dangerous, especially when swept into piles. I am concerned when a small child of mine gets into these piles. I grab her up and rush her to be bathed to get the stuff off her. I want to get away from this. Yet we stay. At one point it seems that to get to this house you have to go down under water. But the house isn't full of water.

I have already pointed out that, in dreams, a house can represent one's body. Here again is mention of a branching growth, this time inside the house, my body. Somehow this growth is coming out of the white dust or moldy growth. I'm concerned that my small child will be harmed by this. A small child in our dreams can represent our hopes and dreams for the future which are growing and developing. Therefore I'm fearful that these might be harmed by the growths which may be representing cancer. At first glance, the last part about having to go down under water to get to the house is more difficult to interpret. But here's a possible meaning. A body of water can represent the unconscious. In order to get into my house to know what is going on there—inside my body—I must go into the unconscious. How can I do that? Through studying my dreams. The message is: "Take note of your dreams, including this one. I'm trying to make you aware that there's a growth inside your body and you should go see a doctor."

I was even given glimpses of what might take place in a hospital more than a year in advance. On Tuesday, August 11, 1992, I dreamed:

Being Examined While on a Hospital Gurney

I am stretched out on what appears to be a hospital gurney. I am told I must stay there. Someone gives me a shot in my side to make me lie still while I am given some kind of physical examination. I don't know why this is being done. But I don't object.

The dream says that "I"—the ego—don't know why this is being done. I am not conscious of what the problem is and why I need to be examined. Too bad I didn't know to take this as a clue to a need to go see the doctor and did not realize I could be helped by healing forces within me.

One of the more amazing precognitive dreams is the one I mentioned at the beginning of this book, the one which occurred on October 3, 1992.

Medical Tests with a Tube Inserted

Others and I are undergoing some kind of "tests" which seem to be medical. We are being anesthetized to have some "tube" or something inserted. This will be left in so the results can be observed and recorded.

At the time, I had no inkling as to what this meant. But, in looking back, I can see now that it was describing the "needle localization biopsy." This method of biopsy is sometimes performed when a suspicious area that shows on a mammogram cannot be felt by touch. As described earlier, after your breast is numbed from a local anesthetic, the radiologist "introduces one or more very fine needles into your breast to the precise site of the abnormality shown on the mammogram. You are then taken to the operating room. The doctor makes an incision in the breast and, guided by the path of the needles, removes the suspicious area." (Quotation from *American Medical Association Complete Guide to Woman's Health.*) In my case, a thin wire was inserted through a tube. The tube was then removed, leaving the wire in place to lead the doctor to the site of the tumor. The entire lump was removed to ensure the removal of all possible cancer cells. The excised tissue was sent to a laboratory to be examined under a microscope.

I also found an earlier dream pointing out my need for self-nurture. On March 29, 1993, I dreamed:

> ***The Kitten Needs Nourishment and Loving Care***
> *I discover a very tiny kitten covered over by papers or other clutter on a table. I realize that this kitten has been there for a long time and has not received any nourishment for days. I marvel at its ability to still be alive and I carefully pick it up, feed and pet it.*

This dream came the night following my attendance at a Mandala workshop given by an art therapist at which an assessment, a guide for understanding one's personality, was made using both the MARI® Card Test© (Mandala Assessment Research Institute) devised by art therapist Joan Kellogg and a Mandala drawing. The drawings placed within a circle were made spontaneously without our being given specific instructions. We could use any color crayons that appealed to us to draw whatever we wished. By studying one's preferences in shapes chosen and colors used in the drawing and test and the placement of such in the drawing, the therapist can learn a person's needs and strengths. I was told my choices showed that there was a part of me that needed nurturing and care and that I needed to see that my own needs are attended to. It's interesting that my dream seemed to echo this evaluation which also corresponds to what I was told by Drs. Sylvest and McLanahan after my cancer diagnosis.

DREAMWORK CONFERENCE AT KANUGA

Even though I had been keeping a dream journal regularly for two years before my diagnosis, I was struggling to understand many of my dreams. Some seemed easy to interpret—at least on one level. Others, as we have seen, were much more puzzling. I was eager to get help both in learning how to interpret and in obtaining some specific input on some dreams. The opportunity to do both came in June of 1994, about two months after the completion of radiation therapy. The Jungian-oriented *Journey into Wholeness* organization was sponsoring a week-long Dreamwork conference at Kanuga Conference Center in Western North Carolina. Although I was still extremely depleted of energy, I was eager to attend.

We had not been to the Kanuga Conference Center near Hendersonville before. I fell in love with the beautiful place. The various buildings are perched on a hill above a small lake and the inn is constructed of stone with wide expanses of window.

The lectures by leading dreamworkers and psychotherapists Julia McAfee, Robert Johnson, and Jeremy Taylor were excellent. For the group dreamwork sessions I chose to attend the ones led by Jeremy Taylor. The group was so large (around twenty-eight or twenty-nine people) that only a few people were able to have their dreams studied. I very much wanted my dream of the fire of burning coals and the fountain interpreted.

On Wednesday afternoon I went to an extra session of a small group which met without Jeremy, thinking I might need to settle on having the dream discussed there. But it didn't work out; they had already decided to work on someone else's dream. I left the session early, feeling anxious and exhausted and needing to rest before supper.

After the evening lecture I spoke to Jeremy, telling him how much I wanted to discuss a dream either with him privately or in the group. At first, he suggested trying the small group. I said I had done just that, without success. He indicated to me that since I had spoken to him about my desire that he would keep me in mind for the group session the next day. I thanked him, and became very hopeful that my wish would be granted.

The next day when I walked into the room where the group meeting was to be held, Jeremy reached out his hand to me and asked if I was ready (or willing, I don't remember which) to have my dream discussed. I was; the session that followed with my dream was an incredible experience, where I both learned a lot and was able to contribute to the group's learning experience.

I shall repeat the dream here along with the possible interpretations which were suggested.

From Burning Coals to a Fountain

I am in a small gathering around something like a campfire with burning coals. I sense that people including small children and other creatures are seeking refuge and protection. I watch and see one or two very small children right by the burning coals. I wonder about their safety. Something (I don't know what) makes me call out urgently: "Get her out! Get her out!" I become terrified and afraid for her safety. As someone reaches for the very small child who is right by the coals she falls over with her head going into the coals. I don't know whether I scream out "She is destroyed" or if I just think this. I don't know if her falling is caused by the person's effort to get to her or if this would have happened anyway. I do not know who it is that reaches for her. But I know no one has done anything quick enough to save her.

I walk up to a place where we are building or preparing to build and I see my father working, constructing a small pool. I don't remember much about the setting. There is no house. But it is outdoors where there is a slight dip in the ground. I see that there is just a small round pool area constructed by the time I am observing. Later I come back and the area is much more developed with some terracing around the pool—as my father often fixed for planting flowers. There is a beautiful fountain with cascading water in the pool.

Interpretation: The "very small female child" who falls into the burning coals is a symbol for the cancer. (In actuality, the cancer was quite small, about the size of a pea.) Just as a child begins with a single cell and grows, so does cancer. When I yell in the dream, "Get her out!", this would mean get the cancer out of my body. The burning coals are symbols for the radiation therapy to be used to destroy the cancer. Therefore the fire, which seems horrible in the dream, is actually what is needed. It has been pointed out that the worst image in a dream turns out to be a picture of the best and most transformative part.

It was also pointed out that persons need to recognize the

attraction of a secret payoff of an illness. What kind of life would I have if the cancer took hold? How would I benefit? Perhaps extra attention and exhibited love would be forthcoming as family and friends help care for me. With a prolonged illness this would continue for the duration. But this is not the "healthiest" way to obtain love. Therefore, for my greatest good in all respects the cancer needed to be killed. (This idea ties in with the suggestion in the discussion of Enneagram Type Twos that persons might become ill due to an unconscious motive of trying to feel loved and cared for.)

> Until the benefits of illness are recognized and alternate means of achieving them worked out, we will not be ready to heal.
>
> — Drs. Michael Greenwood & Pete Nunn,
> *Paradox & Dreaming:*
> *Medicine, Mythology & Transformation*

The cascading water of the fountain was assumed to be a clear fluid, since it was declared beautiful in the dream. Jeremy Taylor felt this to be a symbol for lymph. Therefore, it could have been assumed that there was no cancer in the lymph nodes. The axillary dissection proved this to be true.

If I had known this before my surgery, I might not have chosen the axillary excision of lymph nodes. As it was, at the time I felt I should do everything possible to learn the status of my illness. If I had not had any nodes examined and then later the cancer metastasized, I would have felt I had not done everything possible to prevent it. In reflection, Owen and I have said that it still was wise to have had the axillary excision. Now if I should ever have a reappearance of cancer I will know it is simply a different cancer. I won't blame myself for not doing enough earlier.

My father in the dream could be representative of the Heavenly Father. The dream suggests that God is helping me build a very positive future, with the cascading fountain (the fountain of life) surrounded by terraces for new growth, for planting flowers.

I have had an additional thought since the conference as to who my dream father represents. He could be the inner "wise old man" who can help me build the positive future. He has all the positive attributes my waking-life father had, attributes that I have taken into myself.

Therefore, the entire dream can be seen as positive, showing the means to be rid of the cancer and affirming transformation and new healthy growth.

As this discussion was drawing to a close I felt compelled to briefly tell Jeremy and the group about the series of six dreams that came right after my diagnosis, noting in particular the last one. Here again is that part:

> ***The Man Wants Me to Participate in His Group***
>
> *6. There is a group of people who have participated in the conference and who have been with a particular man in a small discussion group. The man is arranging seats and is either putting name signs on the seats or making a list of people to take part in a future session with him. He sees me and wants to, and, I think, goes ahead and includes me in his group. It seems he wants me to be a part of it. He seems to be choosing people he thinks will be interested and good contributors to the discussions and sessions.*

The experience of participating in this dreamwork session in a way that I felt I was contributing seemed to be a direct fulfillment of this last dream of the "initial series." Breaking into tears, I told the group this. Jeremy very warmly and sincerely agreed.

Several people got involved during the discussion, exhibiting strong personal reactions. Many people hugged me warmly afterwards, thanking me for telling my dreams and recounting my experiences relating to the dreams and cancer. One medical doctor asked if he could have permission to use my experiences anonymously in teaching medical students. I promised to send him a write-up of the dreams and related tales. A counselor asked for the same information and permission. Owen and I, and others attending the sessions, were delighted to think that an M.D. was concerned enough about such matters to be thinking of discussing them with his medical students.

After the conference ended I realized that another one of those "initial dreams" seemed to be foretelling something which happened during the conference week.

I Choose to Stay In and Rest

3. There are various happenings and details related to the meeting (conference) that I don't now remember. One may have to do with meals. One has to do with some people in the group making plans for recreation one evening: to go out and away from the conference place one evening. I think I say I'll just stay there and rest.

One planned event of the conference was an outdoor celebration of the summer solstice after supper one evening that was held around a campfire a short distance from the inn. Since I was extremely tired, still feeling the effects of the radiation therapy, I decided not to attend this festivity, but stayed in my room to rest.

A DIFFICULT DREAM TO INTERPRET

Our dreams, our symptoms, and our sixth and seventh senses [intuition and heart] urge us to discover who we truly are and what we must believe in order to be true to our core self.

— Paula M. Reeves, Ph.D.,
Heart Sense

Some dreams are extremely hard to understand. Some take months or years, if ever, to figure out. It would be very helpful if insights always came as soon as we desire them. It certainly would have helped me. But we need to realize this isn't the way of dreams. We must learn to have patience and respect the natural process of dreams.

The one remaining dream of the "initial dream series" not yet discussed proved to be the hardest to interpret. This one seemed so strange to me at the time I couldn't imagine how it fit into the overall theme of the night's dreams. Many years of additional study of dream interpretation passed before I was able to understand what it was saying. Let's consider it now.

I Dump the Excrement into a Man's Cap

5. I am carrying a container that has excrement in it. I'm not sure whether it is mine or somehow I have collected or picked up some. Any how, I am looking around (outside on open ground) for a place to get rid of it. I see something that looks like a small container on the ground, so I dump the stuff in there. I am surprised to see some man come along looking around on the ground. He seems to touch this object with his lip or mouth as if testing to see if it is what he is looking for. The idea of his doing this repulses me. I certainly think this is strange. He then picks it up and I am either told or realize somehow that the container is his cap. I am very alarmed that I had dumped the shit into it. I think I am apologetic and try to explain what I had done, not realizing the container was a hat. The man doesn't seem concerned. A crowd of people who are around and have seen what is happening actually laugh and/or snicker at the whole incident.

As already mentioned in the section on Self-Nurture, excrement is a waste product from the body, composed of things no longer needed and/or toxins. Inability—in waking life—to get rid of such can lead to physical illness. In the dream, the excrement could be referring to actual lingering cancer cells that need to be eliminated or it could be a symbol for a variety of irritants, negative characteristics, and undesirable aspects of myself which need to be eliminated. These might include negative thoughts and feelings, old hurts, or old habits.

It's interesting to note that "I"—the ego in the dream—am reluctant to claim it as my own. I am ashamed to think it (and what it represents) might be mine. I am also repulsed to think the man has put it to his mouth or lip. Who is this man? On one level he might represent the pathologist who ran the test to check for cancer. But since I think his actions strange (and I wouldn't label a pathologist's actions strange), it is likely there is a important, deeper meaning. I have put the excrement in his cap—perhaps his "thinking cap." Maybe my dreammaker thinks this appropriate as a receptacle for negative feelings and thoughts. A man in a woman's dream often represents the woman's "inner masculine"—the more aggressive aspect of herself that can help the woman take action. By his actions the man affirms that getting rid of the "stuff" is good and he will help me to do it. The crowd of people represent the many extraneous parts of myself that are embarrassed by the whole situation. Snickering is often a sign of embarrassment. The man is not offended and I should not be ashamed or embarrassed.

Remember this dream was part of the "initial dream series." So I was being given advice regarding what I needed to do to "heal" right from the beginning. But at the time I wasn't able to understand this. The dreammaker didn't stop at that point. During the following year other dreams gave the same advice, often in different forms. The dreams in the series including snakes are examples of such. The shedding of snake's skin is a metaphor for shedding old beliefs and negative attributes. Growth for a snake is possible only after shedding the skin. In like manner, our shedding of irritants, toxins, all negative attributes makes possible growth for us, possibly opening up a new path in life, one of discovering one's healing energies and abilities.

Less than two months after completing my treatments, I had a dream which showed activity which I interpret to be the clearing away undesirable irritants, attributes, or attitudes. On June 28,1994, I dreamed:

I Observe Progress in Rejuvenation of My Future Home

I am visiting an old house to which I plan to move. In one of the visits, maybe a second one when I returned alone for another look, I go down into the basement. It's full of muck, mud, silt—mess which needs to be cleaned out before the place is habitable.

In the first visit a lot of furniture is brought into the main part of the house and left. On a later return visit the furniture is still there. I go down into the basement to inspect things. It evidently has been cleaned out some, but is still damp, not pleasant or livable.

On still a later visit, I walk across a ramp bridge to get in. I walk into a room where a small circle of older people, mostly little old ladies (wise women) are. They look up at me, then go on with what they are animatedly discussing. They are somewhat annoyed by my presence, but they don't tell me to leave. After a while they pull themselves into a tighter circle. I stand and watch. I feel I have intruded. Finally I thank them for letting me listen and I slip out.

In the house there is a large living room with a high ceiling. There are very tall windows going all the way to the ceiling, which have arched tops. (I think I'd like such in the new house we are to build in real life. They would let in lots of light, but would be very hard to clean.) In the dream the windows blanket the wall to the outside. The view includes a service station nearby. This is not very esthetically attractive, but I don't mind. It is a part of life.

A house in dreams is a metaphor for the dreamer. The condition of the house, the part of the house we're in, and the circumstances surrounding it give us clues as to its meaning. The house can represent our relationships at home or work, our attitudes, our emotional and mental states, and even our health.

The basement of a house often represents our subconscious mind. But Gillian Holloway in *The Complete Dream Book* states it is much more than that. She believes it is a mixture of psychological storage space and foundational material. "The dream basement, like those in real life, can have numerous and varied functions. This is the psychological space where we file things we have not yet made sense of but which we think might come in handy someday."

In the dream I discover the basement is in bad shape and must be cleaned before it is habitable. So, what old thought patterns and past issues need to be cleared away? How do I need to change my usual way of thinking, believing, and perceiving things? I can be encouraged by three things. One, I have been planning on this move. I'm ready for change—looking to new, revised ideas and states of mind. Second, the living quarters have been furnished and are awaiting my arrival. Third, progress in the cleaning is evident. The tall living room windows with arched tops let in lots of light, therefore much enlightenment is possible. The arched tops bring to mind the spiritual quality of cathedral windows. I don't even mind the view of a service station (a symbol of help). I should give further consideration to the service station visible out the windows. Perhaps this part of the dream is suggesting that if I will look out of the house—beyond myself—I can see a place for—an opportunity for—service.

Many dream basements can reflect the health of the dreamer. On one level the dream is showing that my health is steadily improving at this time. It might also be suggesting that a change in my beliefs and basic approach to certain aspects of my life might be therapeutic. This seems to fit. Several people, including two doctors and a counselor, suggested this might be so.

On my last visit to the house I encounter a group of little old ladies holding an animated discussion in one of the rooms. They are so intent upon their business they pay little attention to me. I think they are "somewhat annoyed by my presence, but they don't tell me to leave. . . . I stand and watch. I feel I have intruded. Finally, I thank them for letting me listen and I slip out."

I consider these women my wise inner feminine council from whom I might learn needed lessons. My ego fears they were annoyed. But since they allowed me to stand and watch, I suspect they hoped I might learn something. I may see evidence of further progress in later dreams.

Sure enough, four years later on March 5, 1998, I again dreamed of renovation of an old house.

> ***I Proudly Watch the Renovation of My Old House***
> *I'm watching construction work taking place in an enormous room in a house. The house is not a new place. I have the impression that it is probably an old place which needs renovation. The room being worked on is the living room with one wall having a large fireplace (maybe made of stones) on the right side (as I am looking at the room). I see a new floor being laid out, made of what looks like rustic logs (squared off) or boards being laid down in a specific pattern. This work has started over by wall on the far side of the room. I believe the person putting down this floor is a woman. I seem to "know" that the house belongs to me. Much activity is taking place. People are coming and*

going, some to do the work, others to see what is going on. I'm pleased with and proud of what is happening.

This time I'm watching the work being done. A beautiful new floor (the symbol of our foundation and basic understanding) is being laid down in the living room in a specific pattern. Thus there is an actual plan being followed to create the foundation upon which I will be living. "I believe the person putting down this floor is a woman." This signifies that my inner feminine is doing the work. "I'm pleased with and proud of what is happening." What wonderful progress is being made.

Then three years later, on March 8, 2001, I dreamed of exploring and discovering all the new additions and changes in our house and yard. I will not recount this dream in detail, but in it there is much activity going on inside and out. Shrubs have been planted in the yard near the building. The style of housing is different; it is a multi-unit place, not a single family home. I discover two people in our part of the building I didn't know were there. Projects are not yet finished. Obviously, many changes are going on within me. More are yet to come; I am discovering new aspects of myself.

TOWARDS TRANSFORMATION

Illness is a call to the transformative potential within us.
We must proceed on our own path, guided by
our own inner healer . . . .

— Drs. Michael Greenwood & Pete Nunn,
Paradox & Dreaming:
Medicine, Mythology & Transformation

Davis Simon points out in *Return to Wellness* that the word "crisis" in Chinese language is formed with the symbols for danger and opportunity. The crisis of cancer can be a life-transforming event that "may yield opportunities for personal growth and wisdom that nourish your body, mind, and spirit in unprecedented ways."

Joseph Campbell, the premier American scholar in mythology who taught for years at Sarah Lawrence College, advises: "Follow your bliss." Many of the countless tales of cancer survivors reveal they have turned their illnesses around, many "beating" their cancer, by "following their bliss." By deciding to allow themselves to do whatever it is they have most wanted to do with their lives, many have lived many years beyond their doctor's prognosis.

Unfortunately, not all cancer patients are cured of their cancer. I have had many friends who have died from cancer in the past several years. But some, although they were not cured, were healed in the deeper sense of the word. There is a difference between "healing" and "curing." In medical terminology one is considered cured when the medical symptoms are eradicated. "To heal" means to make "whole." During their last journey on the earth plane, they grew emotionally, mentally, and spiritually, becoming more fully conscious of their true selves, becoming "whole."

Many people faced with life-threatening diseases ask: Why me? Why now? I didn't ask these questions when the diagnosis was given. But in the years since, I have come to realize these questions are important and should be asked. Why did this illness happen to me? What is the "true cause?" What is the "true purpose" of the illness and why did it come at this time? No one has the definitive answer as to the causes of breast cancer. Many factors enter in. But on one level I needed to become aware of what was going on in my life physically, mentally, emotionally, and spiritually. There are things about my life—my thinking, my understandings, my eating and exercising habits—that need to be changed. The purpose was to call this need to my attention so I can make the changes *now*! This was my wake-up call, a call for transformation.

What does this mean? It is a call to become conscious in the psychological sense in order to become fully the person I am meant to be. My thoughts about the purpose of my life and what I should be doing have taken a different direction ever since.

> A cancer diagnosis can thus lead to a profound transformation of values. Things that used to seem important often become less salient, while other values to which you may have given little thought take priority.
>
> — Michael Lerner,
> *Choices in Healing*

What changes am I called to make? If Vernon Sylvest is correct, I need to nurture myself, care for myself, and quit over-mothering friends and relatives. If Sandra McLanahan is correct, I need to pay attention to diet, supplements, and nurturing my feminine attributes. If the kittens needing care in my dreams represent myself, my inner Self is also telling me I need to nurture myself. How do I do all this? There are many ways which include diet, exercise, meditation, cultivating talents, following my bliss.

I need to consider what "Follow your bliss" means to me. What is it I want most to do? What do I feel called to do?

Although I have been very happy and content with my life as wife and mother, artist and teacher, in the early 1990s (as I have recounted earlier) I began to feel I should be doing something beyond this. But I didn't know what. The uncertainty about what I should be doing was reflected in a dream I had in February of 1992. I dreamed:

I Want to Be Told What to Teach

I am told I have to go back to teaching. This time I am to be teaching in an elementary school. I'm not at all happy about this. When the first day arrives, I still don't know exactly what I am to teach. I meet with the administrators and ask just what am I to teach. Instead of telling me I am to teach "art"—or to teach the ordinary grade work, they simply pick up a brush or some other painting tool and proceed to show me a particular process I am to teach. I feel this is strange and unsatisfactory. I know the process; I feel this is elemental. I want to be told what overall they expect me to teach.

I am told I am to teach in an elementary school—a place of basic learning. I don't think I have been given enough information. I want to know the goal I will be guiding my students toward. I need to know how the process I'm teaching will be or can be applied.

In 1994 I told Vernon Sylvest that I wished I had known years earlier what I know now. He replied that I was not ready for this knowledge earlier. In our early years we do not question the meaning and purpose of our lives. We follow cultural expectations. We learn through our life experiences. Oprah Winfrey—on her June

24, 2000 TV show, *About Us, The Dignity of Children*—made a similar observation: "What we live through is what we become."

I investigated the practice of various alternative therapies: art therapy and mandala assessment, Touch for Health Kinesiology, Therapeutic Touch; and I became a Level II Reike Practitioner, trying to find that special avenue I should travel.

Various people have urged me not to abandon my painting. Joan Windsor told me that my art is important, that viewing a painting can be healing for the viewer. Joan Drescher, a renowned creator of healing art, pointed out in an article in the *Healing Healthcare Network Newsletter* some years ago that a simple image of beauty opens our hearts to hope, helps us heal, and brings forth wholeness. The noted Jungian therapist Marion Woodman said something similar when she stated at a workshop I attended that the images you eat are as important as the food you eat. I do hope that through my art I am helping to provide a nourishing diet, as Marion Woodman suggests, for those who view my paintings. But I have continued my "search" for what more I am called to do.

In 1991, after a lapse of twenty years, I returned to recording my nightly dreams, but without doing much in the way of interpretation. Upon being diagnosed with breast cancer in early 1994, I paid close attention to these dreams and learned that they can offer much healing wisdom. Marc Ian Barasch, in his book *Healing Dreams: Exploring the Dreams That Can Transform Your Life*, states, "I have found that the course of an entire health crisis may be told through dreams, heralding its imminent arrival, providing descriptions of disease processes, bulletins and updates, comments on decisions made, guidance, and repeating themes." I certainly have found this to be true.

In earlier times physicians considered a patient's dreams an indispensable tool in aiding healing. Other cultures share the dreams of the tribe members daily to guide their activities. In Native American traditions a child's dream can reveal his destiny. Unfortunately, in our culture, children are rarely told the value of their dreams. Their parents probably neither understand nor acknowledge their importance. Barasch urges us to wake up to the importance of dreams. Through his own experience he learned that a dream he "had taken to be a psychological refuse heap was a rich archaeological site, awaiting only excavation." He also tells of a former official in the Department of Energy who spends hours each day working on her prolific dreams.

He states that

> she might seem to be literally dreaming her life away. But why shouldn't she so honor her dreams? What would our lives—our very civilization—be like if we considered dreamwork as valuable as our vaunted "productivity"? Perhaps incorporating our dreams into our individual and collective lives would be an ounce of prevention worth a pound of cure, the navigational reading that ensured we were heading true north, not sailing off the edge of the world.

Jeremy Taylor believes dreaming is a spiritual discipline which extends awareness and causes consciousness to evolve. He states that rejection of the deep humanity of our dream experience is immoral. We need to develop language to talk to everyone about these concerns. Survival of the world depends on it.

Dream study and dreamwork have become my "passion." This sounds to me to be the discovery of "my bliss." Quite some time after I first wrote these last two sentences I read *The Bridge to Wholeness: A Feminine Alternative to the Hero Myth* by Jean Benedict Raffa. In it I found a passage that brilliantly describes the meaning of "passion." Raffa writes:

> When one has a passion, one is acted upon by a calling from or to some unknown greater power—a calling that cannot be ignored without endangering one's very soul. . . . Passion, this very feminine quality, is indigenous to human nature and essential for life satisfaction. . . . [L]ike the feminine, it is also life-giving and life-affirming and must be honored in each individual if we are to find the meaning of our lives. Each of us, male and female, needs to learn to find and trust and follow our passion. We need to acquire the necessary self-knowledge of what our passion is, and then we need to develop the courage and discipline to pursue it. The only way we

> will ever feel good about ourselves is by living our lives fully instead of hiding from our true potential. This is the meaning behind Horace's saying, "Carpe diem," or seize the day. It is also what Joseph Campbell meant when he told his students to follow their bliss.

I've read extensively in the field of dreamwork, attended lectures and conferences, completed a two-year study program with the Institute for the Enhancement of Dreamwork and two year-long programs with the Group Dreamwork Training Institute, all grounded in depth psychology and Jungian thought. I spend many hours recording and working with my own dreams. To use Marc Ian Barasch's words, it might seem I am "literally dreaming [my] life away." Perhaps this is my calling and I have found my voice.

On October 13, 2001, I had a dream which seems to suggest this is true.

My Large Cat Speaks

I have acquired a large, full grown cat and have it in my arms in an unidentified location. It seems I'm in some "stranger's" house. Why, I don't recall. The cat leaps out of my arms and races up the stairs. There are some small children in the household who have just been put to bed. Since the cat is new to me, I don't know how it acts with children. I'm worried, fearful the cat might get into their rooms. I call out to warn the adults what has happened. In a minute the man appears with the cat in his arms. He says he was able to catch it easily. He places the cat back in my arms.

I can't remember whether there or at another place later, the cat says a word—literally. I'm startled. So is whoever is there. We make additional conversation and the cat says something—one word—again.

The cat is mature, full grown, no longer a kitten. We are in some stranger's home. There are still aspects of myself I do not know, including children—new, young, undeveloped talents. I'm worried about what the cat might do; I am still unsure of what I am capable of—for good or bad. The man, my masculine attributes from my unconscious, retrieves the cat and places it back in my arms—back under the control of my ego-consciousness. Perhaps the ego wants to keep too much control. Maybe "the cat" should be allowed its freedom to go where it wants. Note that it headed up the stairs to where the children "have just been put to bed." Perhaps this suggests having something to do with dreams, maybe helping children appreciate and understand their dreams. My ego-consciousness and others with me are startled when the cat says a word, then still another. The deep, inner part of me that the cat represents is beginning to speak. It is finding its voice.

While searching through my dreams recently, I was surprised to find a much earlier one in which a cat spoke. On March 2, 1992, I had dreamed:

The Cat Speaks in a Human Voice

We are at our home in a large room. I don't know what the house looks like or where it is. There appears a cat that does not look familiar to us. We wonder whose cat it is. The cat then speaks in a human voice and tells us it is our cat. We are very surprised that it has spoken. We either make a comment or ask a question and it speaks again in reply. I am glad someone is there with me who has heard this—so I know it has happened and might be believed. I think we accept it as our cat. It doesn't speak any more.

It seems that this part of me—perhaps an intuitive part that was already the mature cat—was trying to get my attention long ago, but, as stated in the dream, I didn't recognize it. Although we supposedly accepted it as our cat, I evidently didn't encourage it to express itself. After the initial conversation, "it doesn't speak any more." I found it hard to believe it could speak. I felt other people would find it hard to believe. The ego doubted that people would listen to this part of me. Even though at the time I had already begun to question what new or different direction my life should take, how I could use my talents to help others, it is now obvious I was not ready to make my voice heard.

Now, through facilitating dream groups, one-on-one work

with people, and writing, I hope to teach the importance and appreciation of dreamwork and various ways to interpret and benefit from dreams. Writing might seem to be a new interest, but actually I am returning to the earlier interest. As a ten-year-old child I wrote poetry, several children's short stories which were published in a Methodist periodical, and even a children's book which I illustrated and, with the help of my mother, typed and bound into book form. For the present I have pushed my painting to the side in order to study dreams and write. I don't seem to find time to do both. Somehow I need to find a way to make time, perhaps allocating specific time for each. By doing both I will be giving expression to what I read someone considered "opposite desires of expression: writing and painting; verbal and visual." Doing both can be a way of obtaining a balance of opposites. Also, since dreams are mostly expressed visually, writing about them combines the two forms of expression.

My experience with cancer in many ways seemed unreal; it seemed so strange to be told I had a life-threatening illness when there was nothing I could feel or see and I certainly didn't feel sick. In fact, I felt in most ways healthier than I had ever been most of my life. I did not consciously choose to have cancer. You might think Diane Kennedy Pike had my story in mind when she wrote the following in her fascinating book, *Life as a Waking Dream*:

> Sometimes our life experiences seem almost unreal, as if orchestrated by an unseen composer. We feel caught up in something not of our own choosing, much as we might feel during a dream at night. Those are the very experiences that have the potential to reveal deeper meaning in our lives. As the Russian philosopher P.D. Ouspensky says, "A soul, when it begins to realize that all visible life is but a dream, approaches awakening."

In the last dream of the "initial series" the group discussion leader at a conference is saying I will have something to contribute to the group. As stated earlier, I believe this came true at the Dreamwork Conference I attended soon after completing radiation therapy. I also believe there is an additional meaning. I feel I can continue to contribute in my life beyond the cancer experience in several ways.

By sharing simple images of beauty that I paint, perhaps I can open hearts to hope, help heal, and bring forth wholeness. The same can be done through the sharing of my experience and by helping others learn how to understand their own dreams.

The third dream of September 19, 1995, gave encouragement and advice:

I Have On the Wrong Color Robe

At some point I'm to attend some meeting, or maybe a church service. I have on a black choir robe. I go to a doorway to go in and something is wrong. I'm not sure whether I have come to the wrong door. I think I learn that I have on the robe for the Sunday morning service—or at least a different service (from the one just about to take place)—that the robe for this service is a purple one. I see some people with purple robes on inside the sanctuary.

The dreammaker is saying I should take off the black robe of the unknown, the mysterious, and even the fear of death. I should put on the purple robe of healing abilities and spiritual strength and vitalities, then go join others in the sanctuary for service.

Lord, make me an instrument of thy peace;
where there is hatred, let me sow love;
where there is injury, pardon;
where there is doubt, faith;
where there is despair, hope;
where there is darkness, light;
and where there is sadness, joy.

O Divine Master, grant that I may not so much seek
to be consoled, as to console;
to be understood, as to understand;
to be loved, as to love;
for it is in giving that we receive,
it is is pardoning that we are pardoned, and
it is in dying that we are born to eternal life.

— *St. Francis of Assisi*

Epilogue

I'm not there yet, but I'm closer than I was yesterday.
— Anon

As I approached the completion of the first draft of this book, on Saturday, February 22, 2003, I had the following dream:

I Must Keep Checking the Contents of a Container

There is a cylindrical container kept in an adjacent space behind a closed door. I have been given the responsibility of taking care of this. I'm supposed to check to see when it's time for the contents to come out. I don't believe I know what is in the container to begin with. When I check on it and open the lid, I somehow can tell it is not time for whatever to come out. So I close the lid and leave it where it is. When I check on it later, I see that what is in it has made some effort to move upward. To come out it will need to push its way through a covering at the top which has begun to split open. I see what appears to be the top of a head. The image is similar to that of a baby beginning to push to be born, but the head appears more that of a much older person than a baby. I wonder at what I'm seeing. There doesn't seem to be space in the container for a body with this head. There's nothing I'm supposed to do to help it out; I'm just supposed to check on its progress. Again I leave it and close the door. Quite some time later I remember I'm supposed to keep checking. Since it has been quite a long time since I last checked, I become alarmed. I wonder if I've waited too long and it has died because of my negligence.

My first thought about this dream dealt with the image of something making an effort to move upward. Perhaps this refers to material from the unconscious coming into consciousness. On one level I feel sure this applies. My dreams have been bringing lots of information into consciousness. But I feel it also deals specifically with this book and its completion, when it will see the light of day, when it will be born. Many previous dreams have used the imagery of being pregnant and giving birth in reference to the creation of this book. This dream says that for the contents of the container to come out "it will need to push its way through a covering at the top which has begun to split open. I see what appears to be the top of a head. The image is similar to that of a baby beginning to push to be born." So the time of birth is almost here.

But the puzzle is that there doesn't appear to be space for more than a head in the container. The head is where we process and keep our thoughts; my memories and creative thoughts are what are written down in this book. I have been given the responsibility of caring for the contents of the container for quite some time, even before I knew what was there. The container's round (cylindrical) shape suggests the idea of a *temenos,* which in ancient Greece was thought to be a sacred place where one could find refuge and be safe from harm. This seems appropriate here in my dream. Whatever is in the container is being kept safe until the proper time for it to emerge. I am supposed to keep check on its progress and, I assume, let it out when the time is right. At the end of the dream I'm alarmed, hoping my negligence hasn't caused its death. The answer to that concern is not revealed.

The appearance of an image that was "just a head" caught my attention for another reason. I remembered having dreamed of babies with just heads many years ago. At the time I speculated that the dream was saying that my head was separated from my body—perhaps I was too much in my head. On seeing this new dream, I decided to search for the old one to see how the two might be connected. In the process I discovered two additional dreams. One came in July of 1991, almost eight months before the remembered dream of babies with just heads. I believe the head in this one is an adult, not an infant.

A Head to Care For

I am somewhere, place unidentified. I am meeting some people, strangers that I don't know anything about, and I am asked to go over and care for one particular person, to look after him. When I go there I discover that the person is just a head. There is no body whatsoever. This doesn't seem to be particularly strange to me in the dream. I simply pick up the head and am going to do the caring for it, looking after it. The other circumstances of the dream have escaped me, but that does not seem to matter.

Since all characters in a dream can be considered parts of the dreamer, the people I'm meeting are strangers, parts of myself I do not know. I am meeting and getting to know new parts of myself. Then I'm asked to "go over and care for one particular person, to look after him." This "person" is just a head. On reflection, this seems very strange, but in the dream it "doesn't seem to be particularly strange." The question again might be whether the dream is saying my head is disconnected from my body. For two reasons I don't believe that is its message. One, the head is only one part of the group of strangers I'm meeting. There are many aspects of myself present. Then I'm being asked to take special care of this "head." There doesn't seem to be any criticism or negative connotation involved.

Now I find it amazing to realize I was being asked by my inner being, my dreammaker, my inner Self, to take special care of "the head" over a decade ago—long before I had any notion of writing this book, almost three years before I was diagnosed with breast cancer. I had no idea what this meant. Just two months before having this dream I attended the four-session workshop using mandalas during which I was questioning what direction my life should take, how I could use my talents—my art—to help others. I have described this experience in detail earlier in the book. At the time I was thinking of my "art" as my painting. It would seem that this dream was pointing to a new direction. Now I realize that art can mean much more than just painting; it can include the art of dreamwork and writing.

Then on March 21, 1992 I had a dream of babies with just heads.

Babies with Just Heads

I'm visiting some kind of "child care institution." In one room I find a group of "just heads"—in a row on the floor or on a low level cushioned platform or bench. I wonder how they can be nourished or life sustained with just heads and no bodies to receive the food. I discover that if you lift the heads there are long tubes extending down below them and somehow this makes it okay.

This, indeed, was a strange dream. I had no idea what to make of it. As I have already said, at the time I wondered if it were saying I'm all in my head. Regina Abt in *Dream Child* tells us:

> In folk tales and myths, there are often demonic figures consisting of a head only, or those who are one-legged or one-eyed and so forth; in other words, these figures are incomplete. They represent a one-sided, disfigured human image and illustrate the one-sided and distorted influence of an autonomous complex, overwhelming or taking possession of the ego. . . .

These babies with just heads in my dream certainly are incomplete, but they don't seem to be demonic and they are being cared for in a "child care institution." Maybe dreammaker is simply showing me when the head and what it represents is beginning to be nurtured.

Six years later, November 15, 1998, the adult head reappears.

A Man's Bald Head in a Box

There seems to be some kind of outdoor market place with unusual wares for sale. Some woman is examining small boxes which have what is presumed to be figurines or some objects in them. She, then those around, hear what sounds like a cry from within the box—a cry for help. We begin to think that somehow a small child is inside. She decides to open the box. As she does, we see the head of a bald man seeming to fill the entire small square box. But with the lid open this head pushes up and out and expands into a larger head which is talking to us. I assume there is at least a small body tucked in the box also, but I wonder how this is possible. The person who has opened the box decides she will take it home and care for this "person" (whatever).

Here the head—an adult, bald head—has been boxed in and is crying for help. As the woman opens the box, the "head pushes up and out and expands into a larger head which is talking to us." I do not report what it says, but I can guess that it wanted out of the box. At the time I assumed there must be "at least a small body tucked in the box also, but I wonder how this is possible." Now I feel certain that it was only a head and it wanted out of the box. The woman, one aspect of myself, "decides she will take the head home and care for" it. At the time I was already working on this book, but there was a lot more to be done.

Why have I felt that each of these adult heads has been male? Perhaps because the rational thinking aspect of a personality is often considered to be a masculine attribute. Why would the head be bald? Dreams can exaggerate and distort things to make a point. Even though I did not have to have chemotherapy and therefore did not lose my hair, the head in the dream might be bald to get us to associate it with cancer. There may also be a deeper meaning. Monks and other male religious orders shave their heads as a symbol, signifying the taking of a special vow. The bald head in my dream may be signifying an inner commitment to a spiritual calling which is now coming into consciousness and into public view through the written word. That inner commitment may have been taking shape back in 1991 around the time of the first "Head to Care For" dream. While reviewing additional dreams from the early 1990s I found a dream from Thursday, April 2, 1992, which seems to show this commitment.

I Meet a Very Special Woman

I have gone to a public meeting or gathering with one or two family members. It is in a strange place. I don't remember any specifics. The guest of honor —or guest speaker—is a very special woman, someone such as Mother Teresa. In the dream I know her name. Wish I could remember it now. We are standing or sitting in rows waiting for her arrival. I am on the second or third row from the front. As she arrives, she walks directly towards us. In fact, she comes directly to me, extends her hand to shake my hand, and commends me for having come out to see her. I am very honored. I am the only one to whom she extends this honor. I am dressed with a scarf over my head.

For two reasons I take this gathering to be of spiritual significance. One reason is the presence of the "special woman"—a Mother Teresa figure. The other is the fact that I am wearing a scarf over my head. In some religious traditions for a woman to cover or veil her head is a sign or token of spiritual submission, humility, and reverence. This woman is honoring me by shaking my hand for some reason which is not spelled out in the dream. Perhaps she is aware that I have made a commitment to "service." Or perhaps by coming to see her I am signifying such a commitment. The gathering could even be for the purpose of taking part in some ritual of commitment.

Then three weeks later, on Friday, April 24, 1992, I had a dream which gives a little more information.

I Am to Give a Life-Saving Demo or Lecture to Women

I am with a group of people. Each person has selected something they are supposed to "do." What I choose is somewhat strange. I am to give a demo (not an art demo) or instruction of some kind to women. I believe it is important for me to do whatever it is because it possibly will save lives.

This dream seems to be similar to one I had two months earlier, in February, which I have discussed above. In it I was told I have to go back to teaching, but I was not told what I am to teach. Now in this one I have chosen what I am supposed to "do," but again the subject of my instruction it is not revealed. At least I did not remember when I wrote down the dream. The ego in the dream thinks its choice is "strange." Perhaps at this stage I did not feel qualified; I still had much to learn. The dream does show I have made a commitment, one that was made in the unconscious. "I feel it is important for me to do whatever it is because it possibly will save lives." This indeed is an important spiritual commitment, and it was taking place more than a decade ago.

With the most recent head dream comes the realization that my search for what I should be doing followed an inner plan for me, incorporating a new direction, and now is becoming visible. However, I am still on my "journey"; I have much more to learn. But while I learn, I want to share what I can with others through my writing and painting and work with dreams.

> The healing process not only has a tendency to bring people closer to an appreciation of who they uniquely are and what their unique purpose is in this world. It also brings them closer to God, spirit, inner peace, connectedness, or whatever they choose to call that which is great and mysterious.
>
> — Michael Lerner,
> *Choices in Healing*

Appendix

The complete list of my questions and Dr. Swensson's answers are included for two reasons. First, they will give additional information not included in the summary of our conversation. Second, I feel they might give someone facing a similar situation an idea of how she might compose her own list of questions to ask a doctor she is considering.

1. How much extra tissue would he take out? I planned to tell him Dr. Horsley's recommendation of not taking any further tissue.

Answer: He thinks more should be taken out. He intends to take 1 cm. around the site and including the site.

2. Do you intend to take out lymph nodes? Take a sampling or a dissection?

Answer: He called it an anatonic dissection. He would take out Level I nodes and one-half of Level II nodes, "an axillary vein, two muscles, two intercostal nerves. It will be numb and sting awhile."

3. Are drainage tubes used when taking a sampling? (I may have asked about possible buildup of fluids in the arm afterwards.)

Answer: Yes. Arm fluid buildup is unusual. If axilla is radiated, there is a higher chance of this happening.

4. Radiation - What specific kind would be used?

Answer: Total standard dose.

I asked whether an internal or external beam would be used. I referred to Dr. Horsley's recommendation of taking out only nodes, then giving an extra "boost" to the tumor area. Then I asked what kind of radiation would be used if this were done.

Answer: External - 4,000 units (standard); then 1,000 units boost.

5. Do we need to consult with a radiation therapist now before surgery? After surgery?

Answer: Yes, now—before surgery.

6. Please describe Richard Belgrad.

Answer: Thin and short, balding salt and pepper hair, mustache.

7. If nodes are positive, would chemotherapy be recommended?

Answer: Yes, this would be needed.

I made a note that I wanted to discuss this point further, since my reading told me Tamoxifin is the choice over other chemicals for post-menopausal women.

8. Would this be the hormone tamoxifin or other chemicals?

Answer: Swensson said it would be other chemicals if the nodes were positive. Just what they would be would be decided by an oncologist. Swensson thinks I would probably be given the tamoxifin even if the nodes are *not* positive.

9. Do we need to consult a medical oncologist? Now? After surgery?

Answer: Yes, now okay. It might be good now, but not absolutely necessary. Later probably would be better.

As follow-up I will see Swensson every six months for three years.

10. Would there likely be a different plan of therapy if the node involvement is investigated, thus the axillary operation?

Answer: Yes.

(If the answer had been No, I would have asked: Is there a real need to do this part? I'd rather not have this part of the operation to avoid the possible complications.)

11. During the biopsy, was there any excessive bleeding? I have the feeling that it was taking longer to finish than you first thought it might take.

Answer: It was normal. He was extracting loose breast tissue. Any oozing best be stopped. You have to leave the area absolutely dry.

12. Is there likely a need for a blood transfusion, and therefore would it be good to give some in advance to have on hand?

Answer: No. He has never needed extra blood for a lumpectomy. The nurse said he does not have extra blood waiting because he doesn't expect to need it.

13. Would you be in charge of the follow-up treatment, or who?

Answer: He and others. I would check back to him regularly for certain things immediately. Then I would see him every 6 months for the next three years. There will follow-up with a radiation therapist and/or an oncologist.

14. I commented on being in "good shape" and told him of the past eight months of good nutrition, supplements, exercise, relaxation techniques, meditation, etc. I said I'm working with a good M.D., Sandra McLanahan, on this.

Answer: He said it was always good to know a patient is in good general health when he has to do surgery on him or her.

15. Anesthesia: After telling of my experience of much nausea after knee surgery, which I wanted to avoid this time if possible, I asked: Should I give him or some other person (anesthesiologist) the information of what was used before?

Answer: I should give the anesthesiologist the information. He, the anesthesiologist, will do whatever possible to avoid the nausea and usually can give something that won't cause trouble.

16. Would it be okay for me to listen to tapes with earphones during the surgery?

Answer: He prefers not to have extra wires in the OR. He said I'd be unconscious and wouldn't hear the tapes. I said I understood it was still done some.

17. Date for surgery: I want to wait another week. Any problem? I need to do some things beforehand.

Answer: Okay. Work out the arrangements with Rosa, his secretary.

18. Length of stay in hospital?

Answer: One day, maybe two. I will still have drains in when I leave. In an a.m. admission I will go to a room after the operation.

19. Private room?

Answer: Yes, this will be possible. Dr. Swensson said I would go ahead and be admitted. Rosa said we can request a private room and can get it if available.

20. I may want someone with me during the night. Would there be any problem?

Answer: This will be okay.

21. When to arrive at the hospital for a.m. surgery?

Answer: Arrange this through Rosa, etc.

22. Can you give me the name of someone who has had a lumpectomy with and/or without radiation who would be willing to talk with me?

Answer: Ask Rosa. [She suggested calling Social Services at Johnston-Willis Hospital. Reach for Recovery, maybe, sponsors support groups that meet at Johnston-Willis several times during the week. Women come whenever they can.]

Glossary

Some of these definitions have been quoted and/or adapted from the following references:

James F, Balch, M.D. and Phyllis A. Balch, C.N.C., *Prescription for Nutritional Healing* (Garden City Park, NY: Avery, 1997)

Rudolph Ballentine, M.D., *Radical Healing: Integrating the World's Great Therapeutic Traditions to Create a New Transformative Medicine* (New York: Harmony Books, 1999)

Charles B. Clayman, M.D., ed. *The American Medical Association Encyclopedia of Medicine* (New York: Random House, 1989)

Yashar Hirshaut, M.D., F.A.C.P. and Peter I. Pressman, M.D., F.A.C.S., *Breast Cancer: The Complete Guide* (New York: Bantam Books, 1992)

Susan M. Love, M.D. and Karen Lindsey, *Dr. Susan Love's Breast Book* (Reading, MA: Addison-Wesley, 1991)

Sandra A. McLanahan, M.D. and David L. MaLanahan, M.D., *Surgery and Its Alternatives: How to Make the Right Choices for Your Health* (New York: Kensington Books, 2002)

Michael Murray, N.D. and Joseph Pizzorno, N.D., *Encyclopedia of Natural Medicine* (Rocklin, CA: Prima Publishing, 1997)

allopathic medicine - A term that describes conventional medicine as practiced by a graduate of a medical school or college granting the M.D. degree or D.O. degree.

anesthesiologist - A specialist who administers the drugs that "put you to sleep" during an operation. Anesthesiologists also assess the condition of a patient's heart, lungs, and circulation before he or she is sent into the operating room. They decide what type and how much anesthesia is needed, determine the patient's position on the operating table, watch for signs of trouble, and decide what actions should be taken if an emergency develops.

anima/animus - Archetypal figures of the psyche, as initially defined by psychologist Carl Jung. The anima is the inner feminine attributes of a man; the animus is the inner masculine attributes of a woman.

anatonic dissection - Surgical removal of Level I nodes and one-half of Level II nodes, an axillary vein, two muscles, two intercostal nerves.

aspirate - To withdraw fluid from the body tissue by suction.

axilla - The medical term for the armpit.

axillary dissection - Surgical removal of lymph nodes to prevent recurrence in the armpit and to help decide about follow-up therapy.

acini, lobules, ducts, and lobes - Acini are sacs lined with cells that can produce milk. The acini cluster together to form structures called lobules. The lobules empty into ducts that can carry milk to the nipple. The group of lobules that empty into any one duct is called a lobe. This milk producing system is, of course, not normally activated until childbirth.

blood transfusion - The infusion of large volumes of blood or blood components directly into the bloodstream, done mainly to remedy severe blood loss or to correct anemia.

carcinoma - Any malignant tumor (cancer) arising from cells in the covering surface layer or lining membrane of a body organ. A carcinoma is thus distinguished from a sarcoma, which is a cancer arising in connective tissue, bone, or muscle.

cauterization - A technique used to stop bleeding that involves applying electrical current, a laser beam, or a chemical such as silver nitrate directly to a broken blood vessel.

chemotherapy - The treatment of malignant diseases with certain chemicals.

echinacea - An herbal antibiotic; detoxifies/cleanses blood and lymph and has been documented to enhance white cell activity, thought by some researchers to assist in fighting cancer.

Estring - A vaginal ring that releases estrogens locally into the vagina.

estrogen receptor report - The Hormone Receptor Assay - A test that measures the presence of estrogen and progesterone receptors in the tumor cells. If these receptors are present, the tumor is said to be estrogen-receptor positive or progesterone-receptor positive. These findings have an impact on the planning of post-surgical treatment, since receptor-positive cells are more likely to respond to hormonal therapy.

estrogen and progesterone receptors - Sites on the tumor cell walls to which these hormones attach. Tumors with hormone receptors are more likely to respond to tamoxifen, a medication that blocks these receptors and thereby prevents tumor growth and spread. Such receptors are more commonly present on tumor cells in older women.

external beam radiation therapy – A form of therapy which uses a beam of radiation from a machine outside of the body carefully aimed at the cancer site; usually involves having treatments five days a week for a period of about six weeks.

goldenseal - An herbal antibiotic; detoxifies, removes yellow mucus, clears GI tract of yeast and bacteria; can weaken digestion.

homeopathy - A system of alternative medicine that uses small doses of medicines that would bring on symptoms similar to those of the patient in a healthy person. Homeopathy employs a variety of plant, animal, and mineral substances in very small doses to stimulate the body's natural healing powers and to bring the body back into balance.

hormone replacement therapy - HRT - The use of a synthetic or natural hormone to treat a hormone deficiency. The use of estrogen hormones, sometimes in conjunction with progesterone hormones, to treat symptoms accompanying menopause.

indolent - With respect to the characteristic of cancer, slow moving.

infiltrating cancer - Cancer that can grow beyond its site of origin into neighboring tissue. Infiltrating does not imply that the cancer has already spread outside the breast. Infiltrating has the same meaning as invasive.

infiltrating ductile carcinoma - A form of breast cancer in which "infiltrating" or "invasive" cancer cells have penetrated the membrane that surrounds the duct or lobule.

intercostal - The medical term for between the ribs, as in the intercostal muscles, thin sheets of muscle between each rib that help expand and contract the chest during breathing.

Level I nodes - Lymph nodes located in the breast tissue that extends up toward the axilla (armpit).

Level II nodes - Lymph nodes located just beneath the pectoralis minor muscle.

Level III nodes - Lymph nodes at the apex of the armpit, beyond the pectoralis minor muscle.

linear accelerator - A machine which employs electrical current or generates X-rays and electrons to deliver radiation therapy.

lumpectomy - Surgery to remove the cancerous lump with a small rim of normal tissue around it.

lymph - A milky body fluid that contains lymphocytes (a type of white blood cell), proteins, and fats. Lymph plays an important part in the immune system and in absorbing fats from the intestine.

lymph nodes - Glands found throughout the body that act as a barrier to the spread of infection, destroying or filtering out bacteria before they can pass into the bloodstream.

lymphedema - An abnormal accumulation of lymph in the tissues, causing swelling of a limb. It occurs if lymphatic vessels are blocked, damaged, or removed, resulting in disruption of the normal drainage of lymph.

magnatherm machine - A machine which provides therapeutic heat by sending penetrating electro-magnetic energy deep into the body's tissue. It is used to increase blood flow and metabolic rate, and to improve oxygenation, with minimal skin surface heating. It bolsters the immune system and helps in healing, thus helping prevent the spread of cancer.

mastectomy - Surgical removal of all or part of the breast, often followed by a course of radiation therapy or anticancer drugs.

metastasize - Process by which a malignant tumor spreads from its primary site to other parts of the body.

midsystolic click - Also known as mitral-valve prolapse (MVP), a common heart condition that is, for the most part, harmless. MVP can be present from birth or develop at any age and occurs equally in both men and women.

mucinous (colloid) carcinoma - Cancer cells floating in the mucin, one of a group of nitrogenous substances secreted by a mucous gland. This variant of infiltrating ductal carcinoma of the breast (cancer in the ducts that carry the milk from the lobules–milk glands–to the nipple) tends to occur in older women, is slower growing, and has an excellent prognosis.

naturopathy - A form of alternative medicine based on the principle that disease is due to the accumulation of waste products and toxins in the body, and that symptoms reflect the body's attempt to rid itself of these substances. Practitioners of naturopathy believe that health is maintained by avoiding anything artificial or unnatural in the diet or in the environment. The goal is to produce a healthy body state without the use of drugs by stimulating innate defenses through the use of diet, herbs, and other natural methods and substances.

needle localization biopsy - Procedure in which a needle is inserted into the breast down to the area in question. Mammograms are taken several times during the process to be sure the needle goes to the right place. Next a wire is inserted through the needle. Then the needle is removed, leaving the wire in place to guide the surgeon who will either excise the lump or aspirate it.

neoplasm - A tumor, tissue composed of cells that grow in an abnormal way.

oncologist - A specialist in the diagnosis and treatment of cancer.

pau d'arco - An herb from a South American tree having a long folk history in the treatment of infection and cancer. It contains a compound—lapachol—considered among the most important anititumor agents from plants.

pycnogenol - A bioflavanoid, found in the bark of the maritime pine and in grape seeds; has the ability to neutralize free radicals, aid cell regeneration, and assist DNA cells to reproduce again, and is becoming a valuable aid in fighting many diseases.

primadophilus - A nondairy acidophilus supplement, "friendly" bacteria, that has antifungal properties, helps to reduce blood cholesterol levels, assists in the digestion of proteins, and enhances the absorption of nutrients.

Premarin - A conjugated estrogen product extracted from pregnant mares' urine, commonly prescribed for estrogen replacement therapy to relieve hormonal deficiency symptoms associated with menopause, as well as to prevent osteoporosis and heart disease.

prognosis - A medical assessment of the probable course and outcome of a disease. However, every prognosis is no more than informed guess, and any patient may prove it wrong.

quantrandectomy - Surgical removal of a quarter of the breast.

radiologist, radiotherapist - A physician who is specially trained and certified in the use of X rays, nuclear imaging devices, radioactive substances, ultrasound, and magnetic resonance to see into the body and diagnose and treat problems.

royal jelly - A thick, milky substance that is secreted from glands of young nurse bees, which contains many vitamins, minerals, enzymes, and hormones, and is thought to be useful in treatment of various ailments.

segmental - Breast surgery that takes more tissue than a lumpectomy, but less than a mastectomy.

sentinel node biopsy - Biopsy in which only the "sentinel" lymph nodes, or the first (one to four) nodes draining the tumor and most likely to contain tumor spread if present, are removed. Negative results allow you to avoid most of the objectionable side effects of the standard armpit biopsy procedure. If positive, you may be advised to have the full standard lymph node removal operation to prevent local recurrence and allow more accurate staging.

simulation - Initial process undertaken by the radiologist devoted to accurately determining the area of the breast to be treated. Specially designed equipment, as well as computer technology, is used. The area to be treated is marked with tiny tattoo marks to enable the therapist to reproduce the daily treatment in precisely the same area.

tamoxifen - An anticancer drug used in the treatment of certain types of breast cancer which works by blocking estrogen hormone receptors. It has fewer adverse effects than most anticancer drugs, but may cause hot flashes, nausea, vomiting, swollen ankles, and irregular vaginal bleeding.

temenos - In ancient Greece, was thought to be a sacred place where one could find refuge and be safe from harm.

Bibliography

Abt, Regina, Irmgard Bosch, and Vivienne MacKrell. *Dream Child: Creation and New Life in Dreams of Pregnant Women.* Einsiedeln, Switzerland: Daimon, 2000.

Anderson, Greg. *The Cancer Conqueror: An Incredible Journey to Wellness.* Kansas City: Andrews and McMeel, 1990.

Andrews, Ted. *Animal-Wise: The Spirit Language and Signs of Nature.* Jackson, TN: Dragonhawk Publishing, 1999.

Barasch, Marc Ian. *Healing Dreams: Exploring the Dreams That Can Transform Your Life.* New York: Riverhead Books, 2000.

Barrick, Marilyn C. *Dreams: Exploring the Secrets of Your Soul.* Corwin Springs, MT: Summit University Press, 2001.

Brewster, Barbara Marie. *Journey to Wholeness.* Portland, OR: Four Winds Publishing, 1992.

Burch, Wanda Easter. *She Who Dreams.* Novato, CA: New World Library, 2003.

Cook, John, comp. *The Book of Positive Quotations.* Minneapolis: Fairview Press, 1996.

Crisp, Tony. *Dream Dictionary: An A to Z Guide to Understanding Your Unconscious Mind.* New York: Dell, 2002.

Curtis, Susan and Romy Fraser. *Natural Healing for Women: Caring for Yourself with Herbs, Homeopathy and Essential Oils.* London: Pandora Press, 1992.

Dackman, Linda. *Affirmations, Meditations and Encouragements for Women Living with Breast Cancer.* New York: HarperCollins, 1992.

Dossey, Larry. *Healing Words: The Power of Prayer and the Practice of Medicine.* New York: HarperSanFrancisco, 1993.

Epstein, Nadine, and Rosita Arvigo. "Spiritual Bathing," *Spirituality and Health,* August 2003, 30-31.

Fincher, Susanne F. *Creating Mandalas: For Insight, Healing, and Self-Expression.* Boston & London: Shambhala, 1991.

Fiore, Neil A. *The Road Back to Health: Coping with the Emotional Aspects of Cancer.* Berkeley, CA: Celestial Arts, 1990.

Garfield, Patricia L. *Creative Dreaming: Plan and Control Your Dreams to Develop Creativity, Overcome Fears, Solve Problems, and Create a Better Self.* New York: Simon & Schuster, 1995.

Gibson, Leslie Ann, comp. *The Women's Book of Positive Quotations.* Minneapolis: Fairview Press, 2002.

Greenwood, Michael, and Pete Nunn. *Paradox & Healing: Medicine, Mythology & Transformation,* 2nd ed. Victoria, B.C.: Paradox Publishers, 1992.

Hersoff, Asa. *Homeopathic Remedies: A Quick and Easy Guide to Common Disorders and Their Homeopathic Treatments.* Garden City Park, NY: Avery Publishing Group, 2000.

Holloway, Gilliam. *The Complete Dream Book: Discover What Your Dreams Tell about You and Your Life.* Naperville, IL: Sourcebooks, 2001.

Kidd, Sue Monk. *The Dance of the Dissident Daughter: A Woman's Journey from Christian Tradition to the Sacred Feminine.* New York: HarperSanFrancisco, 2002.

Kradjian, R. M. *Save Yourself from Breast Cancer: Life Choices That Can Help You Reduce the Odds.* New York: Berkley Books, 1994.

Joseph, Barbara. *My Healing from Breast Cancer.* New Canaan, CT: Keats Publishing, 1996.

Lerner, Michael. *Choices in Healing: Integrating the Best of Conventional and Complementary Approaches to Cancer.* Cambridge, MA: MIT Press, 1994.

LeShan, Lawrence. *Cancer as a Turning Point: A Handbook for People with Cancer, Their Families, and Health Professionals.* New York: Penguin Books, 1990.

Levine, Margie. *Surviving Cancer.* New York: Broadway Books, 2001.

McCabe, Vinton. *Let Like Cure Like: The Definitive Guide to the Healing Power of Homeopathy.* New York: St. Martin's Press, 1997.

McLanahan, Sandra A., and David L. MaLanahan. *Surgery and Its Alternatives: How to Make the Right Choices for Your Health.* New York: Kensington Books, 2002.

Moss, Ralph W. *Cancer Therapy: The Independent Guide to Non-Toxic Treatment and Prevention.* New York: Equinox Press, 1992.

Moyers, Bill. *Healing and the Mind.* New York: Broadway Books, 1993.

Pike, Diane Kennedy. *Life as a Waking Dream: How to Explore Your Most Vivid Life Experiences and Find the Meaning Within Them.* New York: Riverhead Books, 1997.

Plant, Jane A. *Your Life in Your Hands: Understanding, Preventing, and Overcoming Breast Cancer.* New York: Thomas Dunne Books, 2001.

Raffa, Jean Benedict. *The Bridge to Wholeness: A Feminine Alternative to the Hero Myth.* San Diego: LuraMedia, 1992.

Reeves, Paula M. *Heart Sense: Unlocking Your Highest Purpose and Deepest Desires.* York Beach, ME: Conari Press, 2003.

Remen, Rachel Naomi. *My Grandfather's Blessings: Stories of Strength, Refuge, and Belonging.* New York: Riverhead Books, 2000.

Risso, Don Richard. *Personality Types: Using the Enneagram for Self-Discovery.* Boston: Houghton Mifflin, 1990.

Rollin, Betty. *First You Cry.* New York: HarperCollins, 1993.

Simon, David. *Return to Wellness: Embracing Body, Mind, and Spirit in the Face of Cancer.* New York: John Wiley & Sons, 1999.

Slater, George R. *Bringing Dreams to Life: Learning to Interpret Your Dreams.* Etobicoke, Ontario: Kingfisher Communications, 1999.

Slupik, Ramona I., ed. and Kathleen Cahill Allison. *Complete Guide to Women's Health: American Medical Association.* New York: Random House, 1996.

Snow, Sheila, and Mali Klein. *Essiac: The Secret of Rene Caisse's Herbal Pharmacy.* Dublin: Gill & Macmillan, 2001.

Soffa, Virginia M. *The Journey Beyond Breast Cancer: From the Personal to the Political, Taking an Active Role in Prevention, Diagnosis, and Your Own Healing.* Rochester, VT: Healing Arts Press, 1994.

Stein, Murray. *Jung's Map of the Soul.* Chicago: Open Court, 1998.

Tanner, Wilda B. *The Mystical Magical Marvelous World of Dreams.* Tahlequah, OK: Sparrow Hawk Press, 1989.

Temoshok, Lydia, and Henry Dreher. *The Type C Connection: The Behavioral Links to Cancer and Your Health.* New York: Random House, 1992.

Thomas, Richard. *The Essiac Report: The True Story of a Canadian Herbal Cancer Remedy and of the Thousands of Lives It Continues to Save.* Los Angeles: Alternative Treatment Information Network, 1993.

Trafford, Angela Passidomo. *The Heroic Path: One Woman's Journey from Cancer to Self-Healing.* Grass Valley, CA: Blue Dolphin Press, 1993.

Wadler, Joyce. *My Breast.* New York: Simon & Schuster, 1992.

Sound Recording:

Woodman, Marion. *Dreams: Language of the Soul.* Boulder, CO: Sounds True Recordings, 1990. 2 cassettes.

About the Author

Rachel Norment facilitates individual and group dreamwork, gives lectures, and writes a newspaper column on dreams. Her training includes a two-year certificate program with the Institute for the Enhancement of Dreamwork and two one-year certificate programs with the Group Dreamwork Training Institute, and many workshops and conferences led by national and international leaders in dreamwork. She is a member of the International Association for the Study of Dreams.

With a B.A. degree in English from Rhodes College and an M.A. in Art Education from the Peabody College of Vanderbilt University, and years of study with leading watercolorists, Rachel has taught second and third grades, arts and crafts in public schools, and drawing and painting on the college level. Privately, she has taught watercolor classes in her studio and painting workshops for art organizations, and has lectured to civic groups. Her paintings have received numerous awards and have been exhibited in many invitational and juried regional and national exhibitions, and may be seen in corporate and private collections throughout the United States. She is a past president and vice-president of the Virginia Watercolor Society, and holds signature membership in the Southern Watercolor Society, Virginia Watercolor Society, Mississippi Watercolor Society, Kentucky Watercolor Society, as well as membership in the Central Virginia Watercolor Guild.

Rachel lives in Charlottesville, Virginia, with her husband of forty-eight years. They have a son and daughter, and a four-year-old grandson.